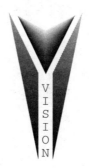

Dedication

For Dori who has always made everything possible

Sex Symbols

Donna Leigh Kile

First published in Great Britain in 1999 by VISION
Paperbacks, a division of Satin Publications Limited.

VISION Paperbacks,
a division of
Satin Publications Limited
20 Queen Anne Street
London W1M 0AY
E-mail: sheenadewan@compuserve.com

Cover Image: ©1999 Nickolai Globe
Layout: Justine Hounam
Photography:
The Kobal Collection
Young & Rubicam
Scott Billups/Electric Sandbox (Virtual Marlon Brando)
Rex Features
Printed and bound by The Bath Press Ltd.

©1999 Donna Leigh-Kile
ISBN: 1-901250-15-6

The Author

Donna Leigh-Kile is an author and freelance journalist who for 15 years has interviewed many major film and TV celebrities in both Britain and the United States for national newspapers and magazines on both sides of the Atlantic, including Life, Parade, US and The Times and Sunday Times of London. She was previously a reporter on the London Evening Standard. She is married with a son, and lives in Surrey, England.

Acknowledgements

I would like to thank Celia Brayfield and Leslie Pound for believing this book was possible, giving me the encouragement to get started and for their support throughout. I also wish to thank the many friends and colleagues who have so generously helped during the work in progress stage, especially Anthony Bales, Andrew Hogg, and Corky Gormly for her succinct and fun questionnaire. Also, Georgina Walsh, Baz Bamigboye, Virginia McKenna, Heidi Kingstone, Liz and Allen Jackson, David Johnson, Rhoda Koenig and in the U.S: Roberta Leigh, David Strada and above all, Dudley Freeman for his invaluable support during those New York years. Warm thanks to: David Mir at Mir-Tech, who technically saved this book; Studio 56's Carol Tilbury and Denise Robinson, Linda Walaszkowski, Jayne Miller, Geoff Norris, Laurette Rice, Rosie Brown, Joyce Attree, Sue Holdsworth, Gary Dobbing and Chris Larkins of Screen Video, Dorking, Linda Butler at Abacab, Dorking, Diane Spranger, Charles Pickstone, Sam Butler, Caroline Bell, Gavin Fuller and Kate Saffett of The Daily Telegraph Library, and to the disbanded Elarose crew whose inspiring leader, Rosina Widmer is so sorely missed.

For the benefit of their professional experience, I want particularly to mention Jeanine Basinger, Margot Waddell, George Butler, Patric Scott, Lindy King, Piers Morgan, Roy Greenslade, Max Clifford, Judy Keshett-Orr, Cary Cooper, Steve Mather, Philip Jones, Bernard Barnett, Scott Billups, and Arianna Stassinopoulos (for an interview about her book The Gods of Greece).

For their time, trust and thoughtfulness I would like to thank all the stars I have interviewed over the years and who are quoted in this book, especially Gillian Anderson.

My fondest gratitude goes to my publisher Peter Hounam for being a very fine friend to have in one's corner.

Above all, my love and thanks to Lowell, Christian, Dolores and Albert whose support and patience enabled me to make this book a reality; and of course, Jamie Leigh who kept me company.

The Cast

The Stars

Gillian Anderson . . . . Actress

Stephanie Beacham . . . . Actress

Michael Douglas . . . . Actor

Mel Gibson* . . . . Actor

Jamie Lee Curtis . . . . Actress

Virginia McKenna . . . . Actress

Barry Manilow . . . . Singer-songwriter

Paul Newman* . . . . Actor

Robert Redford* . . . . Actor

Isabella Rossellini . . . . Actress

Susan Sarandon . . . . Actress

Arnold Schwarzenegger . . . . Actor

Barbra Streisand* . . . . . Actress, singer, film director

Eric Stoltz . . . . Actor

Sigourney Weaver . . . . Actress

Joanne Woodward . . . . Actress

*all quotes in the book apart from those with asterisks are from my own interviews with the cast

The Observers

Baz Bamigboye . Chief Showbusiness correpondent, The London Daily Mail
Jeanine Basinger. . . . . . . Corwin-Fuller Professor of Film Studies at America's
Wesleyan University. . . . . in charge of Clint Eastwood's film archives
Richard Barber . Journalist specialising in celebrity interviews, former editor of
nine national magazines
Scott Billups . . . . Director of Digital Production for Film and TV
Celia Brayfield. . . . . Best-selling Author and Journalist
George Butler. . . . . Film Producer, credited with discovering Arnold
Schwarzenegger
Max Clifford . . . . International Publicist
Dennis Davidson . . . . Head of DDA International Film Publicists
Roy Greenslade . . . . Media Journalist and Commentator
Judy Keshet-Orr . . . . Psycho-Sexual and Relationship Therapist
Lindy King . . . . Actor Ewan McGregor's agent, of Peters, Fraser and Dunlop
Agency, London
Steve Mather. . . . . Former Pop Music Agent turned Lawyer
Piers Morgan. . . . . Editor of the Daily Mirror
Leslie Pound . . . . International Publicist for Paramount Pictures
Patric Scott . . . . Independent Film Publicist

Elsie B. Washington. . . . . Former Editor of the U.S. magazine Essence

*all quotes in the book apart from those with asterisks are from my own inter-
views with the cast

x

Contents

Introduction

S ex symbols are born out of our sexual and romantic hopes and passions, our dreams and desires. Forever unattainable, they are the embodiment of erotic love. They hold the irresistible promise of physical ecstasy through which we can glimpse perfect love, and so we project on to them our very deepest longings for the perfect partner and the perfect relationship.

But our sex symbols are in trouble. Never in their history have they had such high expectations to fulfil. In a culture that views romantic love as the main basis for marriage, our sex symbols are supposed to possess all the qualities that will allow us to fall in love, forever. Forever is the problem. It is incompatible with the impermanent nature of romantic and erotic love. As we have found to our cost, the qualities that make an erotic love object are not those associated with lifetime companionship and raising a family. Yet we expect our sex symbols to reconcile a temporary and essentially ungovernable instinct with 'happily ever after.'

As if that were not difficult enough, we have gone and made our sex symbols human. After all, it has long been recognised that one of the easiest ways to give substance to a fantasy is to lock on to another human image.

In the past, our ancient Greek predecessors believed in gods and goddesses, made in our own human image, who were invested with all aspects of love, and they invented heroes and heroines to illustrate the heaven and hell of our erotic desires. We are still familiar with them today because all sex gods and goddesses in our western civilisation are based on the ancient Greek ideal and are descended from none other than Eros.

The Greeks recognised, as we do, that a sex symbol is a fantasy. But the difference is that in our culture, obsessed with the body beautiful and where the highest premium is placed on personality, we have selected flesh and blood mortals to play this role. What we have effectively done is replace the Greek gods with a human pantheon dominated by movie stars, and relocated Mount Olympus to Hollywood.

This is tough for them, because being human they have a fundamental need to be known, accepted and loved for who they are. But by achieving mythological status they are perceived by their public as glamorised versions of themselves and are constrained by who we think, wish and desire they should be.

Moreover, the demand for human sex symbols comes from a society that is most likely to objectify them and take them for granted. With the industrialisation of sexual fantasy they have become globally available and so easy to manipulate. Assisted by media technology, we have the power to extract the humanity from the being and turn people into products and things at a glance. And we use it. This is why people have such difficulty being sex symbols, or even acknowledging that they are. Being reluctant goes with the job.

Most of the enduring sex symbols of the twentieth century are film stars which is why I have chosen to focus mainly on Hollywood[1] – besides, it's the world I know best, having specialised as a showbusiness journalist in Britain and the US, writing for national newspapers and magazines on both sides of the Atlantic. But the worlds of sport and pop music are also fertile sources of sex symbols because they too produce high profile, charismatic figures onto whom we can project our fantasies.

Sex symbols are a means of releasing sexual energy harmlessly. "They enable us to displace some very strong sexual impulses. By allowing us to fantasise sexually, we don't have to activate that energy," explains US behavioural psychologist Professor Cary Cooper. Thus we are able to walk on the wild side of erotic love courtesy of Richard Gere and Michael Douglas, Madonna and Sharon Stone with all danger, menace and excitement confined to the realms of fantasy.

But there are not enough Connerys and Bardots to go round and so we plug the gap with lesser models – fast food fantasy figures that we treat as one-night stands – easy come, easy go. They should carry a health warning because whilst they may whet the appetite, they can never sate it. In actual fact, they can be addictive.

The truth is that sex symbols lost much of their potent force the moment we made them human. Fantasy figures constrained by flesh and blood are no match for those born of the imagination. Yet no matter how ubiquitous sex symbols have become, we shall always look to them because sex and fantasy are intimately enmeshed with our identity. And we shall continue to place great value on the authentic sex symbols who have managed, against all odds, to hold on to their mystery.

Sex symbols embody our most basic desires and our highest yearnings. But above all, they symbolise bliss however fleeting. For physical ecstasy is the most tangible glimpse most of us will ever experience of that much sought-after, but ever-elusive perfect love.

Sex Symbols

Actor John Malkovich spoke the unspeakable when he defined a Hollywood star as an actor or actress you want to fuck. Considered unfit to print in the British Daily Mail, it does clearly if crudely expose the relationship between sex appeal and box office success.

Sex appeal is an invaluable career asset. But it is an asset that dare not speak its name. While everyone wants to be 'Hot in Hollywood', no one wants to be a sex symbol.

Yet says producer George Butler: "It's the same thing. Usually the casting agents say 'she's hot' or 'he's hot' or 'she's not hot enough for your part.' I'm casting a movie set in Jamaica along the lines of Body Heat, and it's highly sensual. I am looking for a well-known, sexy actress, not only because that is what the part requires, but because that is what it takes for me to get the money to finance the film."

He is competing in a tough market where funding is based on certain known names and demand far outstrips supply. In order to attract them, filmmakers are prepared to pay a high price and so a Hot Name can command sums above and beyond their not-so-hot colleagues.

"It's fascinating to go through the casting lists because they always contain the sexiest actors and actresses," says Butler who is credited with discovering Arnold Schwarzenegger by showcasing him in his documentary film 'Pumping Iron'.

"To name but a few on my list: Uma Thurman, Natasha Richardson, Madeline Stone, Juliette Binoche, Ellen Barkin, Isabella Rossellini, Juliet Ormond and Jennifer Jason Leigh.

"We have been over this list of actresses so many times.

What reaction do they get from the men and, for that matter, the women, we know is the main subject of our discussions.

"The female opinion is very important because it is women who primarily go to the movies, women who influence men to go to the movies with them, and it's women sitting in audiences all over the world paying to see men with sex appeal on the screen. For this reason, when you cast a film an actress will be allocated 20 per cent of the casting budget, and the actor 80 per cent."

But underlying the 'sex sells' commercialism, Butler privately believes there is a fundamental and more covert factor why sex appeal holds such sway in Hollywood.

"Sex is an overriding force in a lot of people's lives, often in a passive and very controlled way. I think it drives people to take jobs or make careers in Hollywood particularly because they are interested in being around great looking women who are sex symbols."

Most of the enduring sex symbols of the twentieth century are Hollywood stars because sex appeal is primarily in the eye of the beholder, and the camera is able to magnify and record for posterity their physical and charismatic attributes.

The invention of the close up has brought the onlooker into greater intimacy with the those on the screen than could be achieved by any lover, who would always have his imagination held in check by the reality of the living person. With the larger than life screen image there is no limit to the imagination's involvement.

According to TV interviewer Clive James, the actors and actresses in close up symbolise the people watching them. "It is a way for the human race to worship itself in ideal form. It happens in public but it is as private as self love,"[1] he writes.

"When Madonna strokes herself on camera she is merely putting her finger on this fact."

The part played by voyeurism cannot be over emphasised. "People love the idea that they can sit in a cinema seat close up to the screen and intimately examine the latest sex symbol, and everything he or she is revealing," says producer George Butler.

But as the relationship is strictly one-way, problems can arise when one projects fantasies and feelings onto an image that cannot respond.

Psycho-sexual and relationship therapist Judy Keshet-Orr explains: "If I project something on to a real person, he can either accept that projection and run with it because it serves a purpose, or he can say, 'I'm not accepting this.' A Hollywood actor or actress can't respond in this way. They are stuck with whatever fantasy we project upon them."

Richard Gere, however, is a fascinating example of a star who has publicly rejected the sex symbol mantle, provoking howls of indignation among the media and even among his fans. How can he dispute it, they argue, when clearly he shows no apparent hesitation or unease at revealing his body or exploring his sexuality on screen? He is noted, after all, for playing highly-charged and erotic roles in films such as *American Gigolo* and *Breathless* and romantic heroes in *An Officer and A Gentleman* and *Pretty Woman*.

But Gere maintains that if he is perceived as sexy it is

only because certain roles demand it of him. Consequently, he will not be defined in any way by his sex appeal. Indeed, when he was introduced as a sex symbol on a British chat show, he insisted it be edited out or he would not do the interview. Gere is damned for denying his sex symbol status but what the hell, he also knows he would be damned if he didn't.

And as it does not fit in with how he sees himself and how he wishes to be seen, he has loudly and actively refused to accept it every step of the way in his career.

Of course, many a sex symbol has railed against the fantasy image that has grown up around them. But Rudolph Valentino is perhaps the ultimate example of illusion overwhelming reality with disastrous consequences. Expected to be the great lover off- as well as on-screen, writes Clive James, he was invested with a god-like sexual potency which elevated him so high, that when he had to undergo an operation no mortal surgeon was thought up to the job. Valentino was not operated on in time, and died.

By the nature of their job, movie and TV stars are ideally placed to act out the quality of sexuality we elect them to embody, and to act as a lightning rod for our feelings about it.

By playing screen heroes and heroines, they get to act out, on our behalf, the themes of love, sex and relationships in visual stories that provide a context for our aspirations and dreams, fears and concerns.

These stories – many based on ancient myths, legends, folk and fairy tales – may be re-worked to suit contemporary tastes and technology. But they continue to be told because although times change, people do not.

A classic case of 'Cinderella updated' is the film *Pretty Woman*, one of the most popular love stories of the 90s. But in keeping with the equality of the era, Prince Charming is transformed by love, too. Richard Gere's character is transformed from a business tycoon with no time to love, and whose fortune is based on asset stripping the companies he takes over, into a tycoon who learns to love, and who pledges to build, not to destroy.

The Pretty Woman played by Julia Roberts changes outwardly from a flashy, cheaply-dressed prostitute to haute couture beauty which dramatically mirrors her inward journey from no self-esteem to self-respect.

The film reinforced Gere's status as a major sex symbol and made Roberts one, because they were the embodiment of what we considered sexy just then. Thus they fulfilled one of the prime functions of a sex symbol – to personify what we regard as sexy and erotic at a particular point in time. Obvious examples today are Leonardo DiCaprio in *Titanic* and Jennifer Anniston in *Friends*.

According to behavioural psychologist Professor Cary Cooper there are two different kinds of sex symbols. One kind exudes a primordial sex appeal, representing a basic biological need. He places Brigitte Bardot and Sean Connery in this class.

The other kind represents the times he or she is living in. Most sex symbols belong in this category. They may simply be physical symbols of their decade or reflect some aspect of our society that we value.

"The Spice Girls represent women's opportunities. They emerged at a time when women were, and still are, trying to push the glass ceiling further up – and became extremely successful in the pop world which had not previously seen many women's groups, let alone success-ful ones."

World-class football players such as the two Davids, Ginola and Beckham also symbolise the aspirations of 90s youth. The girls find them desirable because they are good-looking, young and rich. The boys admire what they do, what they earn and the women they are able to attract and marry.

Former pop music agent turned lawyer, Steve Mather says: "People regard sex symbols or icons as a release from their normal lives. They are a form of escapism. But increasingly they serve an aspirational function. I think we aspire more now because we are bombarded with images and information that encourage us to aspire to all sorts of things – and we have so many more symbols from which to choose.

"An equally important factor is that most people are not satisfied with what they have and so they yearn. If they are have-nots they yearn for something better. If they have everything then they yearn for a bit of rough – what I call the Lady Chatterley and gamekeeper syndrome.

"Most people haven't got what they think film stars or pop musicians have got which is why they set them up as idols. It seems everyone, even Prime Minister Tony Blair, has dreamed of being part of a famous band at some stage, albeit briefly."

Hollywood stars are more likely to attain iconic status because access to them is restricted, says Mather, and when they do emerge they are like Royalty descending –

and then they are gone.

"The key to being a successful sex symbol is not what we know about them but what we don't know and can make up about them. We select our ideal person and then dream subconsciously that they would be like this and behave in a certain way. Because we like them, we also dream that they would probably like us.

"Some of us may hope to meet someone like Sigourney Weaver or Harrison Ford because most of us are naturally romantic and dream a bit – and although we don't consciously think it, these sex symbols may represent our ideal whom we haven't yet met. We don't want to know their faults. We don't want to know that they are fallible or that they wear two pairs of odour eaters in their socks.

"The difference between an actor such as Anthony Hopkins and artistes Rod Stewart and Sam Fox is that Hopkins immerses himself in a character, then switches it on and off accordingly, whereas Stewart and Fox are that personality all the time. It simply expands when they are performing live or in front of a camera. So we only see a very small part of them, the nice bit. But most of us have a dark side that we disguise. And that's the point of sex symbols. We don't want the whole being, for we are seeking perfection.

"I doubt that there would be any sex symbols if people knew what they were really like. I'm sure if Clark Gable took out his false teeth and waved it in front of a group of young girl fans today, the press would pick it up immediately, columnists would lambaste him and in time he would lose his great lover status."

Sex symbols are outward representations of our internal state, or aspirations, or desires which, by their very nature, keep changing. As we change, so do our sex symbols, and in the immortal words of Arnold Schwarzenegger, it's "hasta la vista, baby," and on to the next one.

Their shelf life is, therefore, notoriously short. Sex symbols also tend to be products of their own youth generation and will, at best, remain popular until their admirers grow up, or more usually, until they change allegiance.

Moreover, the expectations of their fickle public are extremely high. Sex symbols today must appear approachable, yet be unattainable; satisfy our voracious appetite for celebrity material but also retain an air of mystery.

As if that were not off-putting enough, US Film Studies Professor Jeanine Basinger, says: "Sex, at one point, was a great mystery, and it had lure and allure. To be a representative of it was a kind of power. That is no longer true. In this day and age sex is readily available, and anything that is readily available is thus devalued and has the potential to be cheap. If you are a sex symbol it is worth less than it ever has been. So, of course, actors and actresses are going to feel diminished.

"Added to which, over history the average sex symbol has been viewed as a tragic figure – just think of Marilyn Monroe and Rita Hayworth – so there is a doom laden quality about it which does not only apply to women.

"Quite apart from James Dean, there were young men such as Montgomery Clift, Tab Hunter, Farley Granger, Troy Donahue, Jim Morrison of *The Doors* and River Phoenix who suffered tragic fates. Furthermore, there is a tendency to over-simplify and forget that there were also teenage male sex symbols who were abandoned as well as female."

This may explain why American agents and publicists are so sensitive about the subject that those approached were not prepared to talk on or off the record.

Or why their British counterparts, and those running international or transatlantic operations (usually British), who did co-operate appear to have such difficulty in even saying the word sex appeal.

"'IT' is a given," says one agent. "Besides more money, those who have 'IT' often get casting approval. This approval is not written into their contracts except in very rare instances, but they do have it anyway.

"This is particularly the case when they agree to be in a small independent film. A director who knows he has a 'catch' is always going to ensure he reaches an agreement about who else is in the cast. On a small budget he doesn't have the luxury of going over and over a scene because the actors are at loggerheads."

One would sympathise with the agents who negotiate their Hot clients' contracts if the process were not so farcical. 'Sshh... you-know-what' appeal must be one of the only commodities that is not actually mentioned when a deal is being struck over it.

Actor Ewan McGregor's agent, Lindy King, has a theory about why she and her clients avoid talking about sex appeal. "There's a kind of superstition surrounding it. Mention it and it may disappear. I think also, that everybody who has it, or is accused of having it is able to call on five or six of their friends who are better looking, who have more success with the opposite sex, and who can pull better than they do. There is always someone else.

"Equally, nobody likes to think they are actually getting work because of it. They like to think that they are getting the role because their work is good, not because they are sexy. You say to an actress that she has huge sex appeal and she will immediately respond that it had nothing to do with her getting the part – She got it because the director thought she was right for it. I've read interviews like that with everybody from Sharon Stone to Madonna. And sometimes it's true.

"But as an agent you send in certain people on certain jobs and you know that if they have gone in at 3pm, at 3.45pm you'll get the call, 'oh my god, they are fantastic,' drool, drool. It's a strange thing, despite sex appeal being such a subjective issue, it's the same names that prompt this response all the time – and not necessarily the most famous ones. Some people have it in spades and you just sit back and watch this immediacy spring up between them and the director and the casting director."

To qualify as a sex symbol one must have a physical magnetism that generates mass appeal. For nearly all women and many men this is inextricably linked to being good-looking, young and possessing a beautiful body. This accounts for the preponderance of sports men and women, film, TV and pop stars, and super models in the sex symbol league.

Their appeal has always been contingent on what they are, not what they do. But the proliferation of supermodel sex symbols today reveals an obsessive preoccupation with image over substance. Actors act, pop stars perform, and sportsmen compete. But as American novelist Jay McInerney has one of his characters say: "Models are the apex of consumer society. Pure image […] I think modern celebrity aspires to the condition of pure image. Modelling is the purest kind of performance, uncomplicated by content."[2]

The exceptions to the physically beautiful ideal are all male and they are to be found in the highest echelons. Jack Nicholson and Gerard Depardieu are classic examples. They demonstrate that men of a certain age who combine talent, presence and charisma can be sex symbols. There is not, and never has been, a female Jack Nicholson or Gerard Depardieu.

This simply reflects real life attitudes towards the opposite sex. A man can be a sex symbol if he makes a woman feel good, and a man feels good by having a beautiful woman on his arm whom he can show off.

Personal power is always sexy in a man; it can be intimidating in a woman. Jeanette Kupferman, the anthropologist who was a specialist adviser on *Yentl*, saw Barbra Streisand struggling with her power as a director.

"Not wanting to be a man was one of the reasons she directed in a very soft-spoken, low-key way. I watched her on the set in England and Czechoslovakia, and at times her direction was so quiet it was scarcely discernible, though there was no doubt that she had total control of everything, from detail on costume to camera style. I told her I noticed this, and she nodded fiercely in agreement, and tried to explain: 'That's the difference, maybe, with being a woman director. I didn't enjoy having all that control. I was embarrassed by so much power.'"

In contrast, Madonna has pushed the boundaries that most women do not wish to broach. Refusing to accept that power and femininity equals masculinity she has managed to maintain her sex symbol status without resorting to keeping the power attached to her appeal hidden or even sheathed. In the sexual arena, her only rival is Mae West who used satire to counter the anti-erotic effect of her power. "I could say almost anything, do almost anything on a stage," West said in her autobiography, "if I smiled and was properly ironic in delivering my dialogue."

Madonna, too, is not averse to using a little irony here and there by throwing contradictory images together – virgins and prayers with erotica and materialism. Nevertheless, says former pop music agent Mather: "Women, generally, feel threatened by the degree that Madonna has succeeded and by the fact that she is comfortable with power which most women are not. It is also extraordinary that her sex symbol reign did not end when she stripped off for that sex coffee-table book. She left nothing to the imagination yet she's still considered a sex symbol."

This probably owes much to timing. Madonna is the embodiment of active female sexuality that has come to the fore in the 1980s and 1990s and which certainly represents the younger female generation, who have not been inculcated since childhood with concepts of femininity which exclude being powerful and effective. Nor do they perceive the cultural image of a powerful woman as an anti-nurturing destructive tyrant or betrayer – a surprisingly pervasive stereotype among their mothers' generation and one that is reflected in the mythology of the female Hollywood star. Actress Faye Dunaway playing domineering Joan Crawford in the clothes hangers scene is a typical example of the stereotype.

Danger, as with power, in a man is often perceived as an aphrodisiac for women. In a woman, post *Fatal Attraction*, it is best confined to actresses like Ellen Barkin whose physical attributes outweigh the risks. A man matures, a woman ages.

Such attitudes have atavistic roots. For despite our common advocacy that sex and reproduction can be considered mutually exclusive, sex appeal at a fundamental level continues to be linked to fertility.

Biologically then, the female sex symbol is at a great disadvantage. Her allure has an allotted life span and she is dependent upon youth and beauty in a way her male counterpart is not. Sean Connery, aged 67, uniquely personifies the male advantage. Huge though his youthful James Bond image remains, it has not engulfed his successive images and he is considered just as sexy now as he was 40 years ago, if not more so – and by women young enough to be his grand-daughters.

As the 'older man' he continues to generate mass sex appeal and retains the title of the world's 'greatest living sex symbol.'

In a recent survey[3] that ranked Hollywood's top 50 stars over the age of 50, on the basis of their ability to get a movie made, the top eight are men.

Besides Connery there is American icon Clint Eastwood, 67, and six major sex symbols, including Harrison Ford, 55, Robert Redford, 60, Jack Nicholson, 61, and Michael Douglas, 53.

In contrast, there are only three female sex symbols Sophia Loren, Susan Sarandon and Goldie Hawn, and they just manage to scrape into the bottom of the top twenty. One consolation is that three former sex symbols qualify, too.

In the midst of all this testosterone, Shirley MacLaine, 64, Anne Bancroft, 66, and Lauren Bacall, 73, show there is professional life and commercial clout after 60.

"Every day you get older. Now that's law." Paul Newman in Butch Cassidy and the Sundance Kid

Ageing, not death, is the arch-enemy of the sex symbol and no star, however well entrenched on Hollywood's Mount Olympus, is immune from the fear of it. They are aware that time will inevitably diminish their looks, their sex appeal and irrevocably rob them of their star status.

As they approach the cut-off point, they worry that they may have begun to look ridiculous in the role of the romantic or sexy lover. For as Burt Lancaster stated boldly, no one wants to see two people of pensionable age making love. At 59, Cary Grant, one of the most popular mature sex symbols in Hollywood history, refused to make the 1963 film Charade until it was guaranteed that he would not be seen on screen trying to seduce Audrey Hepburn, who was more than 25 years his junior.

"He wouldn't do love scenes per se, no kisses," the actress said in 1991, "because he was so much older."[4]

Determined to avoid becoming a caricature of himself, as he saw it, Grant quit acting in 1966, and explained his decision by using an analogy he called 'A Streetcar Named

Aspire.' He says: "In Hollywood we have what I call a 'Streetcar Named Aspire.'

"The thing about this particular streetcar is that it is only so big, and there are only so many seats on it. When I got on, for example, Warner Baxter had to get off. When Tyrone Power got on, Ronald Colman had to get off. And when Gregory Peck got on someone else had to get off.

"Of course some got off more slowly than others and some even ran around to the front and got on again as character actors. Adolphe Menjou was a good example of that. And a few never got off at all, like Clark Gable. Gary Cooper never got off either. He just stuck his long legs out into the aisle and stayed there."

The truth is that it is perhaps only during the closing years of their careers that stars are able to see themselves in their true colours, and can tell if they were really great character actors in disguise (the Alec Guinness type of star), or quintessential Hollywood stars who play themselves perfectly.

Paul Newman confided to his wife Joanne that he dreads being relegated to character parts. "It's very difficult for someone who has had leading man roles, as Paul has had for so long, to give them up and become a character actor," she says. "You get used to being the main star."

At 74, it has yet to happen because Newman has retained his classic good looks, and is one of only a handful of stars whom the public will go and watch, regardless of the film he is in.

He has, in his 70s, convincingly played two love scenes with actresses Melanie Griffiths and Susan Sarandon who are, respectively, more than 30 years, and 20 years his junior. Interestingly, he steered clear of such scenes in his heartthrob years, when his most memorable partner on-screen was undoubtedly Robert Redford.

If such longevity is rare in a male sex symbol, it is unheard of in his female counterpart. "A woman cannot remain a sex symbol, alack and woe, into her 40s. For it is about youth, beauty and let's face it, the body," says film academic Basinger. "Sex appeal in a woman is linked to the power of seduction and so the body is paramount. But in men it is can be partly related to power or prestige or money.

"That's why we have older male sex symbols like Sean Connery and Cary Grant who significantly were not sex symbols when they were very young men."

It certainly explains why the older man-younger woman romantic team is often seen on screen and the older woman-younger man almost never. On the rare occasions it is shown, the relationship is invariably doomed to disaster. Dustin Hoffman and Anne Bancroft in *The Graduate* are an obvious example.

Indeed, the only older woman-younger man partnership that lasted and enthralled the public was to be found, most unexpectedly, in the ballet world. Margot Fonteyn was 40 and considering retirement when Rudolph Nureyev, nearly 20 years her junior became her partner. Their passion on stage, caught forever on camera, captured the world's romantic imagination, and no one gave a damn about the age difference, or even noticed it.

There is no such licence for the jobbing actress, however. Stephanie Beacham, who became a sex symbol because of her 'sophisticated glamour puss' role in the TV series Dynasty, has always viewed acting as a means of raising her two daughters and admits that the physical demands and restrictions on the older actress can pall.

"There's no way that I'm weary of the acting – I love it. But there is a feeling of 'been there and done it.' When I'm working I know I can't go out to dinner, and it's early to bed, because I've actually reached the stage where I have to think about the state of my face. The life of an actress is very self-centred and 'just acting' begins to feel slightly tired. Increasingly, I am open to whatever else is out there."

Living in Malibu, she says, nobody expects her to live up to her femme fatale image which, she says, is not like her at all. "I play devious women and enjoy playing them, but I'm not devious at all. In fact, I'm not really a cat person. I'm actually a good, old, faithful dog."

While the general rule for sex symbols of both sexes seems to be, death preserves and age destroys, Brigitte Bardot is a fascinating exception. For the past 26 years, since she retired from acting, she has made no obvious attempts to maintain her looks and her youth. But such is the power of her sex kitten image that no one who sees her today can look at her without seeing her as she was.

A committed animal campaigner, Bardot gets French government ministers, even presidents to return her calls because they remember her fondly from the film *And God Created Woman* when she lounged on a beach, memorably naked and pouting. "She doesn't act, she exists," said her first husband Roger Vadim, inadvertently summing up her primordial sex appeal.

Her infrequent press appearances are packed with panting media as was recently the case in Scotland where she made a desperate plea for the life of a dog who had the bad, but traditional habit of biting postmen.

Ironically, the sex goddess who attempted suicide three times because she didn't want to "end up decrepit, leaving a negative image of myself" need never have feared such a fate.

Her 1960s image, which continues to exert the same tremendous pull on the 14-16 year old male psyche today, is indelible and timeless, and serves to protect her from ever being seen as she really is.

Footnotes:

1 Taken from Fame in the 20th Century by Clive James published by Random House Inc., New York.

2 Taken from Jay McInerney's novel Model Behaviour published by Bloomsbury 1998.

3 Survey conducted in March-April 1998 by AARP Modern Maturity Magazine. It should be noted that actresses are less globally bankable than actors regardless of age.

4 Taken from People magazine's Special Tribute to Audrey Hepburn issue, January 1993.

Sex Icons

The two sex icons who have had the most impact on our society today are women: Diana, Princess of Wales and Audrey Hepburn.

Sex appeal was hinted at during their lifetime – indicated by Diana's plunging necklines and short hemlines post-divorce, and by Hepburn's carnal kiss in the black and white cult movie, *Roman Holiday,* that stood out because it was in such marked contrast to her innocent Princess role.

But neither of them could ever be accused of overt eroticism. Their physical allure was down to their 'look', which reveals the intimate connection between sex appeal and the fashion industry. Moreover, they represent the attainable body unlike Marilyn Monroe whose natural hour glass statistics remain elusive, and are rarely achieved without the aid of nipping and tucking and some strategically placed silicone.

Princess Diana and Audrey Hepburn shared startling similarities. They were famous for dressing up, able to look perfectly comfortable dripping diamonds or wearing haute couture suits and equally, for their ability to dress down: Diana in blue jeans and white shirt, Hepburn in an all-black outfit – sweater, slacks and shoes. Both were 'wannabe' ballet dancers.

Each developed their own distinctive and instantly recognisable style that transcended fashion and yet was surprisingly easy to copy in parts: the Diana pageboy bob and the ballerina pumps; the Hepburn gamine haircut, the black eye-liner painted lids and thick eyebrows.

Most importantly though, they have come to epitomise thin as sexy, not simply stylish. Not only do they foster emulation and admiration in their own sex but they possess the kind of looks that the opposite sex now finds desirable.

As 22 year old Sam Butler says: "To our generation, the 18 to 25 year olds, we are surprised that Audrey Hepburn was not a sex symbol in her day. I remember seeing a copy of Sky magazine with a copy of Kate Moss on the cover and instantly all the bigger girls at college began to be overlooked. The Claudia Schiffer type was out and we were all talking about the waif look. Since then what blokes have found attractive are very thin bodied girls with pretty faces and Audrey Hepburn is the prototype for those girls and that look."

American Film Studies Professor, Jeanine Basinger observes that Audrey Hepburn is the one movie star from the past with whom her students are able to identify. One senior student went so far as to make a short film about looking for the Audrey Hepburn in herself. "Students here do want to look and be like Audrey Hepburn. They admire her style, sophistication and attainable body, and she seems intelligent. They have respect for the dignity with which she handled her life, her apparent ability not to be eaten up by her Hollywood career, and her humanitarian work with UNICEF. It's partly due to the feminist movement that she has become a sex symbol to our youth. Young men feel they should pick someone like her, and women feel that too. I think it's real. It is the result of having different attitudes about the woman – her role, body and intelligence."

Certainly Hepburn and Diana appeal to the idealistic

side of youth, symbolising as they do compassion. But it is equally their particular brand of vulnerability that has elevated them to icons. Unlike Monroe, whose vulnerability is based on being a victim, they both fought a defiant battle not to become victims. Both suffered from low self-esteem, which manifested itself in anorexia and bulimia that is symptomatic of our times. But it was not so much their suffering that won public sympathy as their determination to overcome it. It also revealed their humanity.

Publicist Max Clifford says: "Princess Diana learnt early on that by manipulating the media she could endear herself to the British and then the world public. Her relationship with the Press and theirs with her was a mutual feeding frenzy, which was hugely successful for both sides. It gave her the strength to stand up to the Royal Family and also made her the biggest star in the world. By being such a huge star she is a sex symbol because she becomes a fantasy."

Many of the indelible images we have of Diana and Hepburn are bejewelled and begowned as befits one who was treated as royalty and the other who actually was, all of which accentuated their separateness. Diana may have been the 'people's princess' but she was still a princess. Being part of a rarefied institution that was unfamiliar with the movie star concept she exemplified, served to isolate her further. But it did enable her to retain a sense of mystery and remain ultimately unknowable, despite playing out so much of her private life in public, and generating an unprecedented amount of world wide media coverage during her lifetime.

Diana beat Hollywood hands down at its own game

because the world was literally her stage and she had access to sets, props and pageantry that the American dream factories could not hope to compete with.

With her sudden death, which resulted in more copy than the assassination of President John F. Kennedy, it became clear just how deeply she had entered the consciousness of the British people. Even those who considered themselves to be disinterested in Diana were taken aback by how personally they took the news and began to realise how much a part of their lives she had become. On the one hand, she was the foremost celebrity in a society where celebrity is a pervasive cult and on the other, she was the enormously privileged underdog who dared take on the royal firm.

"I think that towards the end, they (the royal family) thought Diana was incredibly dangerous," says Piers Morgan, Editor of the British tabloid, The Daily Mirror. "They saw her as a loose cannon capable of anything. Along with the mourning, I suspect, came a sense of relief that she was no longer around to cause the monarchy untold havoc. But her death also changed the monarchy and I think for the good. So if her lasting legacy is a modern thinking monarchy then what a fantastic legacy to leave."

Above all, Princess Diana is a unique media phenomenon that remains addictive even though she is no longer alive to fuel it. That we have become a Diana-dependent nation requiring a regular fix is proved by the millions of copies of newspapers and magazines sold whenever her name is mentioned.

The Daily Mirror interview with Trevor Rees Jones, the

bodyguard badly injured in the car crash that killed Princess Diana is a good example. "We put on 1.3 million papers that week. At 30p a paper, that's a lot of money," says Piers Morgan. "What happened to her was tragic but probably not nearly as tragic as Diana living to 70 when she probably would have become paranoid and miserable.

"She used us and we used her, and the beneficiary in all this was the public who loved her. And they had – I think you are right – an addiction to her that we fed.

"She was the queen of media manipulation. I had quite a lot of dealings with her, which makes nonsense of what her brother said after she died. She probably talked to me more than she talked to him, frankly. The public never knew about most of it, and I didn't feel it was in my interest to tell them because it was all done very quietly. "She would confirm stories, tip me the wink and give me interviews. I would go to the palace for lunch with her and Prince William, and get the low-down on everything that went on. It would come out as 'sources close to the Princess.'

"She obviously had a much deeper relationship with Richard Kay in terms of what she gave him on the The Daily Mail, and there were one or two others dotted around whom she used to talk to as well. We had a very good relationship with her. Then her brother gets up and says we killed her. It was completely ridiculous."

Richard Barber, who has edited nine national magazines and completed a book on Diana's brother, Earl Spencer, says that the British Press behaves the way it does because of the British people.

"You can be sure the proprietors of British newspapers wouldn't put items in their newspapers if the public didn't go out and buy them. In the loosest sense I believe we all contributed to Diana's death, to a greater or lesser extent, didn't we? The paparazzi didn't kill her. What killed her was a man more than three times over the legal drink limit, also on prescription drugs, unable to handle the Mercedes.

"But one of the reasons he was driving too fast was that Diana had acquired the reputation of being the most famous person in the world and was being hounded wherever she went. I am to some extent culpable. People used to ring me up at Woman magazine, screaming at me to take Diana off the cover. This was when we all believed in the Charles and Diana fairytale. I would ignore them. One week I'd do *EastEnders*, the next, Diana – and the sales just went up and up.

"I think she is the ultimate sex symbol this century. There is no male equivalent."

Princess Diana and Audrey Hepburn are icons made flesh – they reconcile unattainability with human warmth. Greta Garbo, however, is more icon than flesh, the embodiment of ideal sex so hopelessly out of reach that all one can do is yearn and sigh in the great tradition of Courtly Love.

Garbo, with her combination of remoteness and perfect classical beauty (impossible to copy) inspired awe because, as celebrity interviewer and author Clive James writes, she 'moved love to the ethereal level for millions of people all over the world who didn't have much time for love on any level. She made them see what they were missing. She did it for them.'[1]

These days, however, we are suspicious of awe. It demands an altogether grander, more operatic scenario – at the very least a pedestal. And isn't that the opposite of what ideal sex is supposed to be about – the ecstatic fusion of two equals? Moreover, there is an underlying fear that while love breeds love, as the saying goes, aloofness breeds obsession.

We prefer charm – it is safer. Natural is better than perfect and slightly flawed is acceptable, sometimes even more interesting. Actor Michael Douglas says: "The screen personas in the days of my father (Kirk Douglas) were truly larger than life. We tend not to be infatuated with matinee idols, either male or female in the same way. All actors and actresses are not regarded as other world beings."

Thus post-Garbo, flawlessly handsome heroes and aloof leading ladies have gradually given way to everyman heroes and heroines.

A most fascinating characteristic displayed by many of our physically beautiful sex icons is their male-femaleness (or androgyny): Greta Garbo and Marlene Dietrich, Valentino and Errol Flynn, all had it. This male-female element is also visible in today's sex symbols: Leonardo DiCaprio, Richard Gere and Tom Cruise have it, as do Sigourney Weaver, Jamie Lee Curtis and Sandra Bullock.

"It makes them more mysterious and interesting, and explains why almost every fabulous looking male movie star is accused of being gay," says film academic Professor Jeanine Basinger. "Perhaps it is related to the old stigma about the actor. If you are an actor you are putting on clothes and make-up and pretending – and isn't that what women do? Obviously, an actress does not have the same problem."

The question mark tends to arise when an actor is a bit pretty or beautiful, not when he is handsome. Nobody says, 'Isn't he gay?' about Clint Eastwood, Liam Neeson or Sean Connery. They have never said it about Paul Newman either, a male beauty if ever there was one. But his long and successful marriage to Joanne Woodward, and aggressively macho image off-screen – he has frequently been photographed auto racing or with a bottle of Budweiser beer in hand – have served to prevent any such thoughts forming.

By embodying some quintessential masculine and feminine quality or qualities of a human being, sex icons appeal to both men and women however ambiguous, or not, their individual sexuality may appear. Moreover, their attraction is timeless even though their image may define an era. Marilyn Monroe, James Dean and the young Elvis Presley truly represent the 50s. Yet they continue to capture the collective popular imagination because they are recognised as the ultimate embodiment of a particular type. Marilyn Monroe is the blonde, James Dean is the teenage rebel and Presley is the rebel rock'n'roller, although there have been, and will always be other blondes and rebels.

All three revealed a unique and instantly recognisable brand of vulnerability, a crucial factor in determining whether one attains iconic status, and in their different ways are viewed as tragic victims. Monroe and Dean swung the sympathy vote by dying young and beautiful. Their deaths were, as Gore Vidal once said of Truman Capote's, a career move of considerable brilliance, possessing all the correct elements for posthumous celebrity: mystery, tragedy, and the kind of aching loss that stars that die violently leave behind.

It is interesting to speculate that by doing so Dean became the rebel icon at the expense of his personal idol Marlon Brando. Brando was an extraordinarily potent sex symbol in his youth who, it has to be said, was infinitely more beautiful, and looked indecently good in levis, white T-shirt and leather bikers' jacket, the trademark rebel gear that is indelibly associated with Dean.

Psychoanalyst Margot Waddell at the Tavistock Clinic, London, believes that what differentiates sex icons from symbols is that the quality they represent and which captures people's imagination is 'set and unchanging.'

"There is no increment of meaning, whereas a sex symbol reflects an individual's changing capacity to find a symbolic representation for an internal state, or aspiration, or desire which may be changing. Symbols are much more linked to internal states that change and develop so the symbols change, too. Icons are timeless because they are not bound in the same way."

The unchanging nature of the Hollywood sex icon is reinforced by the recycling of their familiar image. The re-releasing of universally popular films, and the sale and reproduction of publicity photographs and bills and posters advertising hit films from yesteryear, are instrumental in perpetuating the cinematic legend.

One should not, however, underestimate the power of

being a legend in the first place. "Marilyn Monroe is a sex symbol to me and my friends, now. Her aura is that she is so hugely famous. There can be few men who cannot conjure up her poster image. She has the legend behind her," says 16 year old Morgan Floyd-Walker.

And what a difference that can make is amply demonstrated by film director Michael Winner. 42 years after Winner wrote a film review slating Monroe's performance in *Gentlemen Prefer Blondes*, he paid £3,450 for a 1950s publicity photograph of her.

"Because she was blonde and had sizeable bosoms I assumed she was of no importance," he confessed. "The same prejudices exist today – but not in me."[2]

The year before he had been outbid for a signed photo of Monroe which eventually sold for £8000.[3] Record prices were also paid for her sex symbol clothes, raising the question of the part played by fetishism in the celebrity market. The Monroe strapless, full-length, black silk evening dress fetched £2,070 and a pair of her trademark stiletto-heeled shoes circa 1952 made £1,610.

The images of Monroe, Dean and Presley are so ubiquitous – they decorate everything from carpets and cups to Burger King walls and bedroom closets – that it hardly matters whether one has seen their movies or not.

Ironically, Betty Grable, who is the only female star in US film history to last ten consecutive years in the top ten box office draw, is an icon because of a single image – not her movies. The pin-up photo of Grable looking over her shoulder and showing off her million dollar legs (insured via Lloyd's of London) is evocative of the Second World War.

But the appeal of most Hollywood icons is sustained by showing their films to each new generation and, naturally, the more popular the film, the more potent the icon.

The sex appeal exuded by Clark Gable as Rhett Butler in *Gone with the Wind* and Sean Connery as the original James Bond still seduces mass audiences today. The way they were is considered sexy now, added to which both actors define the sexuality of a particular era, the 40s and 60s respectively.

Thus they exemplify the chief characteristics of an icon. Their sex appeal transcends time but their image as Rhett and Bond are fixed in our collective memory: Gable sweeping Scarlett up the grand staircase to the bedroom; Connery brandishing a smoking gun, surrounded by a bevy of bikini-clad Bond girls.

ICONIC IMAGES AND CINEMATIC MOMENTS

1920s:
Rudolph Valentino dressed as a Sheik
America's sweetheart, Mary Pickford with her head full of golden curls
1930s:
The face of Garbo
Jean Harlow bathing in a barrel in *Red Dust*
Clark Gable as Rhett in *Gone With the Wind*/Gable sweeping Scarlett up the grand staircase
1940s:
Betty Grable looking over her shoulder and showing off her legs, insured by Lloyds of London for $1 million, epitomises the US version of the 'forces sweetheart' in the Second World War.

Humphrey Bogart in *Casablanca*, in trench coat and snap-brim hat, also in white tuxedo and black tie, smoking a cigarette.
Rita Hayworth as Gilda, shaking back her hair, in the 'Are you decent?' scene

1950s:
Marilyn Monroe, keeping cool by standing over a subway vent, with dress blowing up in *The Seven Year Itch*
James Dean in t-shirt and jeans, with hotrods/also, with rifle across his shoulder in *Rebel Without a Cause*
Elvis Presley, hair quiffed and greased, swivel hips encased in jeans
Burt Lancaster and Deborah Kerr in the beach kiss *From Here To Eternity*

1960s:
Brigitte Bardot in a bikini/topless
Sean Connery as *James Bond*
Ursula Andress rising out of the ocean in *Dr. No*
Raquel Welch as fur-clad cave woman in *One Million Years B.C.*
Audrey Hepburn, sophisticated in black, holding a champagne glass in one hand, and stroking a cat with the other in *Breakfast at Tiffany's*
Anne Bancroft pulling on her stockings watched by *The Graduate* Dustin Hoffman
Cooler King Steve McQueen in *The Great Escape* trying to jump the barbed wire fence on a motor bike
Clint Eastwood in *For a Few Dollars More* as the poncho clad Man with No Name, chewing on a cheroot

1970s:
Clint Eastwood as *Dirty Harry*/John Travolta dancing in cream suit in Saturday Night Fever
Paul Newman and Robert Redford as *Butch* and *Sundance*

Sly Stallone running to the top of the steps in *Rocky*

1980s:

Terminator Arnold Schwarzenegger in 'hasta la vista, baby' mode

Officer and Gentleman Richard Gere in his white officer's naval uniform sweeping the heroine off her feet in a factory

1990s:

only time will tell. Possibly Leonardo DiCaprio and Kate Winslet, arms outstretched, standing on the prow of the *Titanic*.

Footnotes:

1 Taken from Fame in the 20th Century by Clive James published by Random House, New York.

2 Taken from the Evening Standard 19.9.96

3 See appendix to find out the record sums raised by film posters.

Sex Objects

Pamela Anderson and the pin-up signify a coming of age for objects of desire.

As the ultimate babe in *Bay Watch*, the most watched TV series ever, she has been lusted after by countless millions of viewers in 110 countries round the world. By reason of her long blonde, perfectly toned bikini-clad image being instantly and globally recognisable, she should surely have qualified as a sex symbol. Shouldn't she?

But ironically, the sheer ubiquity of her image has worked against her. It has made her an object. The very teenagers who pinned up Pamela Anderson posters on their bedroom walls in the early – mid 1990s, also, it seems, had the most contempt for her. She became too available. And as with anything that is in great abundance, it is held cheap. As one 15 year old said disparagingly: "She's just a body to me."

Fame, which usually endows its recipients with a unique starry identity that separates them from the crowd, has had the opposite effect on Pamela Anderson. In her case, her identity as an individual has been entirely consumed in her more general function as an object of sexual desire.

Unlike her pneumatic Playboy predecessors she is not anonymous. But her success, just like theirs, has been based on the sexual stereotype of woman in a decorative but passive role, somehow always less than the sum of her body parts.

The pin-up was originally, of course, based on the same premise: the female as the passively receptive object of the masculine gaze. But in the quest for equality of desire, women soon revealed that they, too, were capable of ogling the opposite sex – as Chippendales' proved with the launch of their striptease evenings for hen parties in the 1979, and Cosmopolitan magazine with its male nude spreads.

Women generally remain wary of sex objects in the flesh and like them to keep a certain distance. Chippendales recognised this when they moved their act from a club venue to the stage. Carol Tilbury, of the Studio 56 Beauty Centre in Beare Green, Surrey speaks for many of her sex when she says: "I suppose we imagine them the way men imagine female sex objects – as dumb blondes without any sort of education. It's probably not true but it's simply the way we perceive them, which is partly why I wouldn't want anything to do with them. I would be embarrassed to see the Chippendales at a club. I wouldn't want them coming right up to me. There's no place to hide."

Her colleague Linda Walaskowski adds: "Because a Chippendale is an object rather than a symbol no personality is involved, and because of what he does there is no desire to get to know him and find out what type of person he is. In the theatre as opposed to a club we, the audience, are the active, threatening ones. We are in control."

Predictably, the advertising world was quick to target this new market. The graphic posters for Calvin Klein briefs, 'lumps, bumps, an all' broke new ground but it was the Diet Coke commercial in the mid-nineties that capitalised on the female desire to actively and publicly lust by actually depicting it.

The ad shows a group of female office workers stopping work, and rushing to the window at the same time each day, to catch sight of a hunky builder pulling off his shirt and knocking back his drink. This action titillates the spectators who fall into a mass swoon. Moreover, women TV viewers have said that registering the female interest in this way enhanced the hunk's sex appeal in their own eyes.

Women, of all ages and backgrounds, are exercising their personal power by doing what men traditionally have always done. They are objectifying the opposite sex. Male babes are the result, and there is clearly an ever-expanding strand of women in our culture who are enjoying babedom for all it's worth.

The popularity of prime time TV shows like *Man oh Man*, in which male babes have to show how well they kiss, move, and look in their bare essentials, before a live audience of 450 screaming and wolf-whistling women, is an obvious example.

The contestants do not see themselves as exploited, or demeaned by the experience which entails being filmed doing press-ups in their swimming trunks, and being pushed into a swimming pool by a female celebrity guest if they are eliminated. Rather they regard their objectification as a career opportunity. By appearing on national TV, they might be spotted by a talent scout or agent.

One winner, actor Sam Butler says: "I thought – what a break. During the selection process I was asked if I would take my shirt off – would I sing? Yes, yes, was the answer. Honestly, I can't see any harm in wearing trunks on national TV and singing a song – and that was as low as it was going to go."

But he admits: "I was the first contestant out and the audience horrified me. Most of them were between 17 and 25 and when I faced them they shouted and swore, and I thought if they had had bricks, they probably would have thrown them at some point. In the final round I found it difficult to hear what the celebrities were asking me because hundreds of girls were screaming.

"It was clear that they thought I was 'cute.' But what help is cute in a show that is basically about how good your body is, how big your packet is in a pair of tight shorts, and do they fancy you?"

By making a pass at the girl with glasses and kissing her a la Valentino, Butler's 'cute' won over raw sexuality, demonstrating against all odds that charm can seduce even the most hostile female audience.

Journalist and best selling author Celia Brayfield observes: "It is now accepted that girls will be girls. They will scream at male strippers, they will wolf-whistle men in the streets, and they will go out, get legless and be silly. This shows that the active principle in female sexuality has to be something that society now basically accepts."

The Hollywood embodiment of the 1990s predatory sexy female is, of course, Sharon Stone who, according to Baz Bamigboye, chief show business correspondent of the London Daily Mail, developed this image on the advice of her American publicist in an effort to get more work.

"Stone was told she had to get out there and do what nobody else was doing and that was to symbolise 90s sex, which is all about up front sex, easy access and glamour. Her timing was perfect. When Marlene Dietrich died, Stone was in Cannes and she said that Dietrich was an enduring benchmark for glamour, allure and complicated sexuality. Stone went on to identify with those actresses who had a hard edge on screen like Barbara Stanwyck and Bette Davis. Davis wasn't beautiful but she had the power to hypnotise and keep you looking at her. She was a bad girl getting away with it until the very end."

Stone's popularity coincides with the emergence of the laddette whose behaviour may manifest itself in an aggressive, loud-mouthed, even destructive way and the equally in-your-face attitude adopted by a new breed of sex objects who are all in favour of the babe boom. It is not only lucrative to be a successful babe but now that it is no longer automatically equated with bimbo, it has become acceptable.

In our society, which is so visually aware, good looks are at a premium if combined with the right amount of personality, intelligence, or talent and ambition. The 90s babes recognise this and actively exploit their face, body and sex appeal as valuable commodities.

'Babe' reputedly owes its currency to the 1988 film *Bill and Ted's Excellent Adventure*, in which Keanu Reeves applied it to any female who passed the 'phworr test'. More than a decade later it is used everywhere.

There are:

The Rock and Pop babes, Natalie Imbruglia, Björk and Alanis Morissette who in interview after interview have set the ground rules. Imbruglia insisted on wearing a heavy winter coat throughout a photo shoot for the Sunday Times Style section (no doubt causing consternation for a magazine that is not accustomed to running cover-up features).

The Trust Fund babes such as Tara Palmer-Tomkinson and Tamara Beckwith who are happy to sell their refinement to promote Kentucky Fried Chicken, or in Beckwith's case, to pose nude save for handbag and a pair of Blahniks.

The Action babes, articulate ballet dancer Sylvie Guillem, and Helen O'Reilly who besides earning £100,000 a year as the Gladiator Panther from the LWT show and its spin-offs, set up a health club and a clothing-distribution company with her husband. Two years ago, the couple moved into their new £500,000 home which they bought outright.

The Media babes, Denise Van Outen, Ulrika Jonsson, and the two Zoes; Ball, TV and radio presenter, and Heller, newspaper columnist.

And, of course, The Movie babes, with Alicia Silverstone who, having started her own production company aged 19, rating as one of the most confident.

Treating sex appeal as a commodity and actively capitalising upon it is by no means the preserve of the babes. Sex symbols have been getting in on the act, too. One has only to refer to Cosmopolitan's '100 Sexiest Men Alive' supplement enclosed with the magazine's 25th anniversary issue.

The men deemed most desirable are almost exclusively those who have received the most TV and movie exposure. This reveals the strong links between sex appeal, fame and box office pull, and inevitably maximum magazine exposure is given to those males who expose the most. Lots of chests – a surprisingly high number of them hairy – are flaunted, emphasised by a macho array of buckles, belts and vests. Does the bald male fear – and find – a strong correlation between hirsute and sexy?

As for the intimate revelations from some of Cosmo's chosen 100, they are so toe-curlingly trite that they make the much-derided Miss World contestants seem like intellectuals in comparison.

"I well up whenever the puppy appears on the Andrex commercials." Trojan the gladiator aka Mark Griffin.

"I clip my nasal hair." Tim Vincent, ex-Blue Peter presenter.

"I wear Vitapoint cream in my hair – the stuff grannies use – to stop it fluffing up into an Afro. Singer and song writer Stephen Jones.

"I've got a flower tattooed on my right foot, and the Converse All Star boot logo on my ankle." British ballet dancer William Trevitt.

And if there were a prize for the bad sex quote it would be split between actors, Stephen Dorff: "I'm young and crazy and a hormonal psychopath for beautiful women." And Jean-Marc Barr: "When I see a beautiful woman, I can't turn it off (his sexuality). I love women. I trust emotion more than I trust control."

Clearly, sex as a commodity has become so pervasive that the distinction between sex symbol and sex object is in danger of disappearing altogether. The babes, male and female, personify the blurring of the line.

Sex objects no longer accept that they are victims. They are as complicit in normalising their own objectification as their audience, by insisting that they are in control, and in Cosmo lingo, rulers of their own destiny.

They have, grammatically speaking, made the transition from passive to active objects – and the active voice says: 'It's okay for me to objectify me. But it's exploitation if anyone else tries to capitalise on my assets.'

Once upon a time in the twenties, to be an 'It' girl meant that one possessed it – sex appeal. Today, if one is an 'It' babe – male or female – one runs the very real risk of being viewed strictly as a commodity and becoming It.

The difference between a sex symbol such as Sharon Stone and celebrity sex objects in general is not merely to do with degrees of fame or sex appeal or talent, but that the latter present a more accessible fantasy. They say, "This could be you/yours" while Stone, for all her overt sexuality, says, "Only in your dreams."

Sex objects who become celebrities are in an extremely vulnerable position. They lose the protection guaranteed by anonymity but fail to achieve the degree of safe separation between themselves and their public that is usually accorded sex symbol stars who are perceived as ultimately unattainable.

The Pamela Anderson-Tommy Lee private "honeymoon tape" that wound up on the Internet is a cautionary tale for sex objects operating in today's market place, where there exists a voracious consumer demand for surveillance-reality video, focusing on celebrity and sex.

The Internet Entertainment Group's creator Seth Warshavsky who was responsible for putting the tape on the Net (it was sent to him by a TV producer) said: 'The second we got it, we decided to put it on the Net. We reviewed the legal history and the legal status of the tape.

We were very comfortable about running with it. It was phenomenal – It basically doubled our business.'[1] The tape went out on a network of sex sites that wanted to license it. After Anderson and Lee failed in their legal attempts to stop the tape's distribution, they gave Warshavsky permission to sell the video. It enabled him to earn $15 million last year and the 25 year old mogul claims it is the best-selling adult video in history.

Moreover, his company is to release the collectors' edition of the tape. According to Warshavsky this contains 30 per cent more sex and he expects to sell in similar numbers. The reason why the Pamela Anderson and Tommy Lee video sold so well is, he said, 'because you're looking at the lives of a rock star and a movie star in their real surroundings, what they're really like.'[2]

The Anderson-Lee sex video raises more than the issue of whether or not we should allow Net porn businesses to pander to our worst voyeuristic tendencies at the expense of celebrities' privacy.

There is also the pernicious premise that it's okay to publicise the tape because Anderson and Lee have built their careers by exploiting their sexuality and have, therefore, forfeited any right to privacy in their personal lives.

International film publicist Dennis Davidson says: "I think it is quite scary. It's an interesting comment on people's lives that many of them have to live vicariously through someone else. I have a real problem with the invasion of privacy. I personally don't believe that I, as a consumer of the media, have a god-given right to the intimate details of people's lives just because they are celebrities."

Sex objects have always had a notoriously short shelf life but today we are able consume and discard fantasy figures with unprecedented speed, owing to the 'now' communications technology which enables us to access their images immediately wherever, whenever.

This has had a devastating impact on the career span of many pop performers as former agent turned lawyer Steve Mather explains. "I used to send clients past their prime to Russia, the Far East and India because then they didn't have satellite TV and were probably ten years behind in terms of musical tastes. But now that you have Indian MTV, for instance, full of break dancers wearing turbans and baggy pants, the market no longer exists and so such bands and singers get left behind and are forgotten."

Global technology has resulted in a certain homogeneity of who and what we consider to be sexually attractive images of Pamela Anderson and Harrison Ford are as appreciated in Estonia and Lebanon as they are in Europe and the US. But it is possible for an individual to have more than one image and be perceived differently in different countries.

The common image we have of Samantha Fox in Britain is as The Sun topless Page Three pin-up. But in the US, where she had three top ten records in the Billboard charts and a successful first album in the 1980's, and throughout the former USSR, Japan, Europe, Africa and Australia she is known as a pop star, having sold more than 20 million records. Indeed, in India she topped the bill over Duran Duran, which took the group aback.

Mather, her agent for four years, says: "Her recording

career started first but her father sold her page three photographs on the back of it before I started representing her. It is true, however, that her sex appeal had a lot to do with her success. She was perceived as singer and somebody who was obviously very sexy with her clothes on. In England, however, we have never allowed her to be anything more than a Page Three topless model and her records did not sell at all well here."

Fox's career, launched when she was 15 years old, illustrates the problems and insecurities that can arise from being publicly objectified. From the beginning everyone, it seems, wanted a piece of her. First there was her father who abused her trust by mismanaging her business affairs, leaving her to face a tax bill she could not afford to pay despite her worldwide income.

Named as one of the 200 richest women in the UK by the London Sunday Times, Fox was in an invidious position. She wanted to preserve her status and establish her credibility – she was set to buy the house next door to Margaret Thatcher in London's Dulwich Village – yet she also needed to work to pay off her debts and raise money for the court case against her father.

Mather, who was brought in by her accountants, says: "It's difficult to say 'I'm available for work' when everyone thinks you are rich and play golf all day. The recording situation was a problem.

"We put out a greatest hits album to establish a profile because once you are out of the public eye as a pop performer people forget about you, especially if you are a teenybopper singer. There's always somebody younger and fresher to take your place. Unless you are a credible artist you can't have a long silence, you've got to be there.

"My job was to find places where she could work and earn a lot of money but where nobody in the media would be bothered to check up on her – places like Urengoy, the Milton Keynes of Siberia, Riga, Latvia, Lithuania and India. What she was desperate to avoid, and equally as her agent what I wanted her to avoid, was the public saying that she was trying to earn a few bob before everyone forgets who she is.

"A major concern in some of these technologically unsophisticated countries is the increased likelihood of damaging photographic images arising. If, like Sam, you are known for your looks then photos of you looking your worst – in your curlers, or taken at an odd angle so you appear to have a double chin, or with your make up running, because of the stage lighting – are at a premium."

Which brings us to the quintessential problem faced by sex objects. They are the basic measure against which their own sex judges itself in terms of their physical appeal to the opposite sex. Women, knowing that Fox is considered sexy by men, and whilst comparing their attributes with hers, tend to be critical or dismissive if not openly hostile towards her.

Mather observes: "When we were out in South Africa the all-women crew were initially determined not to like her. They were suspicious of her probably because she was obviously what men liked and perhaps they felt they were not up to that.

"They all wanted to see if she had had her boobs done or whether her body had been nipped or tucked. There was a curiosity based on mistrust and I suppose an element of jealousy as well. In Sam's case she was so used to living the image, like a pop star, that she actually found it very difficult not to be like that.

"Nonetheless, by the end of the two weeks the women crew had changed their minds and admitted liking her. This was interesting because in my view while both men and women appreciate a sex symbol, a sex object is usually only appreciated by the opposite sex."

One can only surmise that the crew's working engagement with Fox was time enough for them to see beyond the image and view her as a woman whom they actually liked, rather than just an object.

Having to contend with an automatic bias against her by women, Fox also faced being regarded as a trophy girlfriend by the opposite sex. "She had boyfriends but none of the relationships were long lasting and the odd thing is that I think she was quite lonely," Mather recalls. "She was surrounded by drooling guys who told her she looked fantastic and was marvellous because she needed to hear that. But they were doing it for one reason only, I'm sure, and that was to get into bed with her.

"Most of the blokes I saw her with I could never see her marrying. Half of her wanted to settle down and have kids like her mum but her image was always getting in the way. Whenever we went out in north London she would walk around in a baseball cap and didn't wear make-up because she didn't want to be recognised. She lived alone and already had problems with people coming to her door.

"She was absolutely desperate for reassurance. She needed people who were willing to give her 24 hours and tell her every second she looked wonderful. She didn't want the reality.

"It's understandable because most artists like that feel they have always to look their best because that's what their public expects of them. A spot or zit wouldn't matter to you or me but to them it's a disaster because people are scrutinising them whatever they are doing. They are terribly insecure and there seems to be no way out of it. I think of all the sex symbols I have met and frankly they are all very unhappy people."

The commodification of sex appeal risks de-humanising not only established sex objects and sex symbols but any personality or celebrity who colludes with the sexy way of selling and marketing him or herself. Whether one is the President's wife and actively agrees to appear on the cover of American Vogue or becomes a sex object by association as in the case of Monica Lewinsky, our response to them is the same. We comment on their weight and judge them on their looks, their make up and their clothes. Substance disappears as soon as they become a two-dimensional image.

Footnotes:
1 taken from *Life* The Observer Magazine 7.2.99
2 ibid 2

Sex Symbol Archetypes

In our western civilisation, today's sex symbols may all be one hundred per cent human, but they can legitimately claim to be descended from an illustrious and immortal family tree.[1] For what we have done in the twentieth century is replace their Olympian ancestors with a pantheon dominated by movie stars, and relocate Mount Olympus to Hollywood.

Whoever the sex idol; Leonardo DiCaprio or Sharon Stone, Harrison Ford or Cameron Diaz, he or she conforms to at least one of a limited number of archetypes defined by the classical Greeks, and embodied by their gods and goddesses, demi-gods, and mortal heroes and heroines.

On the face of it, Richard Gere and Jack Nicholson would appear to have little in common apart from their mass sex appeal. But these two stars happen to belong to the same archetype – they are Snake Charmers. Meg Ryan's beauty may be diametrically opposite to that of Julia Roberts, nonetheless they too share the same archetype. Both of them are Sweethearts.

Supreme deity is, of course, Sean Connery. Having pumped iron, then loved, seduced, fought, rebelled and roguishly charmed his way through seventy films, he has, in his forty year long career, encompassed all the male archetypes so many times. Even premier league sex symbols Kim Basinger and Kevin Costner are left breathless: "He's such a specimen of maleness," Basinger says.

"With the film *The Untouchables* he himself became untouchable when everyone realised what a fantastic film actor he was [...] Sean Connery probably is the biggest star in the world," says Costner.[2]

Sean Connery is The Great Unknockable. Nobody wants

49

to have a go at him; least of all, the notoriously sniping British tabloid press who would fall over each other to give him copy approval.

Yet this one-time Adonis, now Zeus-style commander-in-chief does admit to an Achilles heel. Constantly voted the world's sexiest man, he remains at a complete loss as to an appropriate verbal response. Well aware that any comment could easily be construed as false modesty on the one hand and an inflated ego on the other, he lets his physical trademarks do the talking: one quizzically raised left eye brow followed by the Connery smile (mouth and eyes incorporated). Combined, they give him the appearance of sharing a confidence with each one of his worldwide audience, personally.

If Connery is considered a god by Hollywood and ripe for canonisation by his native Scotland, then The Unknockables: Paul Newman, Clint Eastwood and Robert Redford are demi-gods. As are Muhammad Ali, The Ultimate Fighter, and Liz Taylor, Sophia Loren, and Tina Turner, who are the foremost Ultimate Divas.

All of them were supremely beautiful in their youth and by surviving, in some cases even defying physical age, and overcoming personal tragedy, suffering and illness in varying degrees, they are unconditionally adored by their public, and have become unassailable.

Their reputations, fortified by myth and legend, are impervious to mortal attack. Rumour, malicious gossip, even the truth are either metamorphosed and then absorbed into their fortress-like image, or simply ignored as if they had never existed.

This élite reigns over a sexually magnetic and highly

charged hierarchy:

The Divas first. Their classical Greek ancestor would have it no other way. Aphrodite, the goddess of erotic love and beauty (Venus to the Romans) was completely irresistible to all mortal men and her fellow gods, including Zeus. Only the three Olympian virgins were immune to her power.

The Divas are the femmes fatales of the family. Through their roles, these actresses reflect the two sides of the Aphrodite archetype – the dark as well as the bright side. Sharon Stone in *Basic Instinct* and Michelle Pfeiffer as Catwoman drive men and Batman to distraction with their power-games, treacheries and sheer erotic beauty. They remind us that Aphrodite was also known as 'the dark one' and 'the killer of men.' As one Renaissance philosopher-turned-tortured-soul, warned: 'Only Venus [Aphrodite] comes openly as your friend, and is secretly your enemy [...] She promises you her deadly pleasures and promises more than she ever delivers...'[3]

In the twentieth century where such a high premium is placed on reason, it is clear that Aphrodite in this guise is our very worst nightmare. The movie *Fatal Attraction* touched a raw nerve when it showed how easily lust and desire are able to overpower rationality and common sense, and then depicted in frightening detail the dire consequences.

Yet the other side of this love goddess – free-loving, uninhibited and naturally sexy – has fuelled countless male fantasies throughout the ages. One has only to think of the iconic image of Marilyn Monroe pushing down her billowing dress in *The Seven year Itch* to see why.

This 'golden,' 'glowing' archetype, as described by the ancient Greeks, has had many other Hollywood incarnations since Monroe: the youthful Brigitte Bardot; Jane Fonda; Julie Christie; Raquel Welch and Ursula Andress, to name but a few. Indeed, when Andress steps out of the sea onto a sandy beach in the first Bond movie, *Dr. No*, it is none other than a cinematic version of Botticelli's painting, Birth of Venus. Both the Cubby Broccoli and Botticelli sex goddesses emerge from the sea barefooted, long-haired and gloriously unselfconscious, complete with shells. The main difference is that Venus rides the waves on her scallop shell while Andress carries hers.

Aphrodite au naturelle may be her most seductive and popular look today but she is also the goddess of glamour, and the cosmetics and perfume industries; in fact anyone or anything connected with the arts that enhance beauty and love-making. Liz Taylor, because of her turbulent private life rather than any acting role, *Cleopatra* included, is undoubtedly the supreme example of glamorous Aphrodite. Eva Peron is also a contender.

As for heavenly Aphrodite, well, she has always been extremely rare as the human race, in general, has never really got to grips with the concept of ethereal sex. Yet ironically one of the greatest Hollywood sex icons of all time embodies this archetype: Greta Garbo. The name given to her, the Divine, denotes her unearthly beauty, sublime sex appeal and absolute unattainability.

There was no-one like her before, and the odds are heavily stacked against any of today's sex symbols joining her because our society has effectively thrown away their pedestals.

Thus all our divas conform to the five remaining principal Aphrodite types:

Earth Divas: Susan Sarandon, Ellen Barkin, Jessica Lange and Isabella Rossellini.

Prime example, Sophia Loren.

Fire Divas: Whitney Houston, Uma Thurman, Sean Young and Nicole Kidman.

Prime example, Rita Hayworth.

Ice Divas: Kidman (again), Gwyneth Paltrow and Kristin Scott Thomas.

Prime examples, Catherine Deneuve and Princess Grace.

Air Divas: Michelle Pfeiffer, Darcy Bussell

Prime example, Audrey Hepburn

Supermodel Divas: Caprice Bourret, Eva Herzigova, Claudia Schiffer, Naomi Campbell.

Prime example, Lauren Hutton.

The Ultimate Divas either encompass several types such as Tina Turner, or one superlatively well, i.e., Sophia Loren as Fire Diva.

The Divas motto could equally be interpreted as a warning: 'Bewitch, bother and bewilder.'

Ares the god of war was certainly bewitched, bothered and bewildered. He was so passionately in love with Aphrodite that everywhere she went so did he. Their relationship demonstrated the link between love and war and sex and aggression that remains a familiar juxtaposition today. In twentieth century terminology, it is known as a love-hate relationship.

As the embodiment of aggression, strife and turbulent love, Ares in Hollywood terms amounts to big box office. Our most celebrated male stars, Sean Connery and The Unknockables included, have all embodied this archetype as Action Men or Rebels and Rogues many times during their career.

Mel Gibson in Mad Max and the *Lethal Weapon* films; Harrison Ford in *Star Wars*, *Blade Runner* and *Indiana Jones* and Tom Cruise in *Top Gun* and *Mission Impossible* portray the positive aspects of this blockbuster force that fuels the 'American Dream'. They embody rugged individualism, the drive to win, making it against all the odds and the spirit of adventure.

Many of the action movie stars are also Swashbucklers. By dint of their epic adventures, wanderings and romantic encounters, they become hero adventurers and thus conform to the Odysseus archetype. Odysseus was a classic Greek human hero who, after fighting the Trojan War, which lasted ten years, spent another ten years trying to get home, battling a myriad of fantastic enemies with which producer George Lucas and his special effects department would have a field day.

Besides the Action Men, two other types come under the Ares archetype:

Great Sports, such as tennis player Andre Agassi, soccer players David Beckham and Michael Owen, and basketball player Michael Jordan. On a league of his own, however, is Muhammad Ali, The Ultimate Fighter.

The final type, the Rebels and Rogues, encompasses the negative as well as positive attributes of this archetype. Kevin Costner as *Robin Hood*, Clint Eastwood as *Dirty*

Harry and Paul Newman in almost everything epitomise the hero rebel and outlaw, whereas Warren Beatty in *Bonnie and Clyde* and John Travolta in *Pulp Fiction* reveal the destructive underside of rebellion and mindless aggression.

George Clooney in *ER* and Brad Pitt in *Legends of the Fall* are the acceptable face of roguery; Sean Penn in *The Game* and Billy Zane in *Titanic* show us its unacceptable side.

Clint Eastwood's catch phrase 'Make my day,' would be an apt motto for this archetype.

Eros, according to late Greek myths, was born of Ares' and Aphrodite's passion, which represented a great loss of face since he started off as the oldest god whose realm spanned 'the endless space of heavens to the dark abyss of hell.'[5] And the decline did not end there. Eros is now reduced to Cupid, the cute cherub piercing the hearts of lovers with little pin-prick arrows.

As far as Hollywood is concerned, however, what Eros lost in primordial power has been amply replaced by financial profit. For The Sweethearts embody this archetype.

They are the Mr and Miss Nice Guys of Hollywood and the men in particular epitomise the seductiveness of humour to the opposite sex, which more than compensates for their lack of conventional beauty (in Dudley Moore's case, also his lack of inches).

The supreme and most successful example of this type is Tom Hanks whose very niceness has been held against him. Critics, at a loss to find anything to criticise, accuse him of being too nice. As one carping interviewer said:

'Nice, nice, nice, nice, nice,' which as everyone knows is four nices too many and rates as a nasty putdown. Having achieved overwhelming kudos and fame in the 1994 *Forrest Gump*, he has resisted the urge to give free reign to his ego in an industry where, according to film correspondent Tom Shone, stars' egos have their own trailers.

Hanks' relationship to his own fame is something of a marvel, he writes: 'I'd give it four levels of sophistication beyond the normal: he is a) ironic and self-deprecating, all the time being aware of b) the dangerous point where self-deprecation shades into false modesty, and so seeks to dispel a hint of c) lil-ole-me disingenuousness with d) frank, up-front and unironic acknowledgements of that fame.' What saves the male sweethearts from being sickly sweet or too bland is their tart comedic observation that, in Hanks and Steve Martin's case, is compounded by the physicality of their humour.

Martin especially, seduces the opposite sex both with his throwaway verbal wit and easy dancer's motion that has a sophistication not seen since Fred Astaire. A man who can make a woman laugh, and move like that too cannot possibly fail as demonstrated in the film *Roxanne*.

As the re-incarnated *Cyrano de Bergerac*, Martin succeeds in winning the love of the beautiful heroine played by Daryl Hannah because of how he made her feel: 'romantic, intelligent and feminine.' But neither he nor the film lapse into sentimentality – his humour sees to that – and Roxanne ends with two jokes, not a kiss.

His and Hanks' underlying looniness surfaces in Robin Williams, the third and final example of a male sweetheart.

He proves that if you talk fast, furiously and funnily for long enough you may not win the girl on screen but you will be loved by your audiences.

Julia Roberts, Sandra Bullock and Meg Ryan, all Sweethearts, are three of the most bankable female stars in the world.[4] Their name on a movie is considered a virtual guarantee of substantial box office returns.

Roberts, who is currently the highest paid actress in Hollywood, having agreed to team up again with Richard Gere and *Pretty Woman* director Gary Marshall, well and truly demonstrates the commercial clout this archetype commands.

But perhaps the ultimate sweethearts dream team comprises Tom Hanks and Meg Ryan, who with the 1993 film *Sleepless in Seattle* to their credit, have this year collaborated in *You've Got Mail* in which they play bitter rivals who fall in love through their email exchanges. A major theme concerns their perceptions of each other and how they differ online and in reality.

Without exception all the screen sweethearts are far more complex, sharper and tougher than their screen personas will admit. The boy and girl next door may be nice but they should not be underestimated. Hollywood has never made that mistake. Doris Day, the sweetheart icon, would be proud of her successors.

Their motto: Sugar and Spice.

Ironically, it is Doris Day who struck a major blow for TomBoy women when she played the swaggering sharpshooter Calamity Jane in the 1953 musical of the same name.

While she was willing to be 'feminised' – wear a dress and perfume – unlike her cowgirl predecessors, she refused to give up her superiority with a gun to win her man.[5] By the end of the movie, she is wearing the pants again, still out shooting any man alive, with admiring cowboy husband predicting an 'exciting' future together.

Tomboy women conform to the Artemis archetype, the androgynous and freedom-loving goddess of dance, hunting and wild things.

Passive femininity has been swapped for an active 'in your face' approach, and overt fleshy curves have been traded in for high performance, muscularly sculpted bodies (breasts naturally enhanced by toned pectorals), able to hunt down and eradicate aliens in Sigourney Weaver's case, or world destroying humanoids in Linda Hamilton's. Self-confessed Tomboy off and on screen, Jamie Lee Curtis, who actually played an ex-Olympian turned aerobics teacher in the film *Perfect*, observed that most men like her tomboy look but dislike the glitzy, high-glamour photographs taken of her.

Artemis is also the western model for the modern career woman: independent, powerful, and aerobically fit. It is an image that has driven women into gyms, leggings and trainers – and made Jane Fonda a fortune. Their motto: Don't fence me in.

If Artemis embodies contemporary woman, then her twin brother Apollo is the Hollywood ideal of leading man. All the most physically beautiful actors and athletes conform to this archetype: the young Muhammad Ali, Marlon Brando, Clint Eastwood, and Robert Redford; Paul

Newman and Sean Connery still; Michael Jordan, Tom Cruise, Mel Gibson, Kevin Costner and Richard Gere.

By satisfying a deep human longing for flawless beauty, this group has the greatest commercial clout, the best chance of an enduring career, and the highest earning potential of any sex symbol archetype. It also possesses the highest number of prime candidates for overwhelming fame.

Two of the most bankable stars in the world embody this Apollo archetype. Tom Cruise, who has a hundred per cent rating, and Mel Gibson can guarantee an up-front film sale regardless of the script, cast, producer or director brought to the package. Their names alone assure studios of a strong opening weekend for these stars' films.[6]

But their popularity is not based on looks and form alone. Apollo is the god of truth and justice and therefore these male beauties are credited with brains, ability and heroic roles to match. Denzel Washington and Michael Jordan are not simply supernovas in their respective fields, they are also held up as role models. This is the least likely group to be heard complaining that they are not taken seriously. Their motto: Speak true, right wrong. Else, wherefore born?[7]

The Apollos typically graduate from the Adonis junior league. Adonis was a supremely beautiful youth who despite his mortality proved irresistible even to the love goddess Aphrodite, who described him as 'thrice fairer than myself.'

Her passionate adoration of him would no doubt be understood by the millions of school and teenage girls who worship Leonardo DiCaprio, the most celebrated and commercially successful Adonis of our times. Such was his appeal in the film *Titanic* that it was estimated that his young female audience returned to see him at least four times on average, and 30-40 times in extreme cases.

Just how much of the $1.793 billion so far generated by the blockbuster is accountable to his presence has been the subject of much speculation – maybe as much as half of that billion dollars.

While this is unprovable, DiCaprio, on the strength of his last three films, *Romeo and Juliet*, *Titanic* and *The Man in the Iron Mask*, is able to command $25 million a picture, $5 million more than Tom Cruise. It would not be surprising if he looked bemused by his impact when one considers DiCaprio is only 23 years old. He has six biographies already out, and he is at the top of the International Star Chart published by Screen International Magazine in September (1998), way ahead of every established sex symbol in the business.

The question is, will he be able to make the transition to Apollo status where he will be assured a long and lucrative acting life? Tom Cruise made it and Brad Pitt is almost there because of their canny choice of roles. But the pressures in the Adonis league are unprecedented. When the teen audience is not being obsessive it is fickle and an Adonis can find himself being burned by overwhelming fame one minute, and dumped and forgotten the next. Whichever situation, his youthful inexperience is a disadvantage and burn out is all too common. While the spotlight remains on him, however, the Adonis motto is: 'Youth will be served.'[8]

Unlike the modern media that seems strangely perplexed by the DiCaprio/Adonis phenomenon (if nothing else it is an indication of just how middle-aged and male-dominated the mass media still is) the classical Greeks would have thought it perfectly natural. After all, the emphasis on the male body comes from them and it seems they were the first to make representations of naked male youths as images of ideal beauty. Known as kouroi, they were not so much cult statues as dedications or offerings at a god's shrine.[9] No, what the ancient Greeks would find inexplicable is the vastly increased status of Hebe, the goddess of female youth. In their day she was a dull, lesser deity whose sole claim to mythological fame was her marriage to Herakles, better known as Hercules, the strongest man in the world. Centuries later she was resurrected and revamped by the fashion, film and TV industries to re-emerge as the most dominant, desirable and potentially dangerous archetype of western society today, that of the girl-woman. Hebe's descendants are the Millennium Eves and the Waifs and Strays embodied by the likes of Cameron Diaz, Uma Thurman, Gwyneth Paltrow and Kate Moss. It is this look that causes girls as young as nine to question their shape, teenagers to diet, starve themselves and, in extreme cases, even die for the look and women to undergo plastic surgery so as to maintain maximum youthfulness. For adult female beauty is now commonly defined as being as girlish as possible – Goldie Hawn epitomises the mature girl-woman as did Felicity Kendal in the British sitcom *The Good Life*.

But it is Audrey Hepburn above all who embodies the

Hebe archetype. Consequently, although she was not considered a sex symbol during her career, she has become a sex icon since her death.

She is regarded as one of the classiest pin-ups among middle class males aged between 18 and 25. As she observed in her lifetime, 'the truth is, I know I have more sex appeal on the tip of my nose than many women have in their entire bodies. It doesn't stand out a mile, but it is there.' [10]

As Hepburn's black and white films attain cult status among a generation who were not alive when they were made, she has been vindicated. The motto of this archetype is: 'You can never be too thin.'

Muscle men have always had a role to play in Hollywood but until the advent of Arnold Schwarzenegger and Sylvester Stallone they were considered dumb-bells. Usually relegated to 'punch first, think never' gangster/bodyguard roles, the rare few who did attain leading man status found themselves playing Biblical strong men like Samson or variations on the missing link. Johnny Weissmuller as Tarzan springs immediately to mind.

But Schwarzenegger is credited with overturning this dumb-bell image and thus re-instating the Hercules archetype to its former heroic position. Capitalising on his bodybuilding background he has, through sheer personality, astute choice of roles and a self marketing genius, demonstrated that muscles can be smart, sexy and in his case, extremely profitable. According to George Butler, producer of the 1977 film *Pumping Iron* that made

Schwarzenegger famous, the star is largely responsible for making muscles a prerequisite of the ideal Hollywood body.

"After Arnold appeared in 1972, Richard Gere, Jeff Bridges and every actor of any note started going to the gym. It's true of actresses too."

With the *Terminator* and *Rocky* series of films, actors Schwarzenegger and Stallone have elevated the status of the Pumping Iron archetype to a level not seen since classical Greek times when Hercules, regarded as a legendary hero, was described as 'the greatest man that ever lived on earth.'[11]

Their motto: 'The triumphant conviction of strength.'[12]

Hercules together with some of the best known Greek heroes, Jason, Achilles and above all, Odysseus were protected, advised and guided by Athena, battle goddess of education and science and the most powerful divinity after Zeus. Born from Zeus' head, fully armed and independent, she is completely at home with the masculine order and demonstrates that action, power and intellectual creation are as natural to a woman as a man. Of all the female archetypes this is the one least likely to provoke envy or jealousy among women. For if there is a politically correct type of sex symbol then Athena is it: the thinking woman's ideal of a thinking sex symbol who has taken and translated masculine power to serve her own purposes.

This archetype is equally popular with men who find the Athena-type intelligence appealing because it is, well, so male. Men can identify with the rationality, political persuasion, pragmatism and ruthless militant action, characteristics they have long associated with their own sex, and they value what Athena represents: law, justice and politics, all traditionally male areas. This is a goddess they can do business with, the answer to Professor Higgins' chauvinist plea in the musical *My Fair Lady*: 'Why can't a woman be more like a man?'

Above all, the Athena archetype is the promise of the ideal female companion who is on the same wavelength as her man. Here, at last, is a woman he can understand but who is, as her own sex recognises, cleverer than her man. Sigourney Weaver is Hollywood's prime example of the Brains and Brawn beauty.

But it is perhaps Gillian Anderson as Agent Scully in *The X-Files* who epitomises this archetype. Analytical, scientifically sceptical and unflinchingly brave, her sensibility is disguised by layers of common sense, and her figure impenetrable under those bulky, drab suits and coats.

This mind and body cover-up allows audiences to read whatever they like into her inscrutable face, from unresolved sexual tension to love, with the result that Gillian Anderson has been voted the sexiest woman on TV several times, much to her bemusement.

"To me Scully is anti-sexy, almost. That was why I did do a publicity jump at one point to try and get the audience and the people in the business to understand that Agent Scully was not me. I wanted to show another side of myself, that there was an opposite inside, something a little more lively and sexier. So I did the cover of FHM magazine. I didn't do many other sexy covers like that but

I have done a lot of covers – it's a creative outlet for me – and sometimes they come out as sexy but that is not the intention," she says.

The irony is that by playing the only truly mysterious female character on TV, Anderson actually owes her sex symbol status to what she does not reveal.

The Athena motto: 'United we stand, divided we fall.'

Hermes the winged god of transformation was the cleverest and most complex of all the gods. He was able to bridge the gap between god and man, life and death, commerce and the intangible realities of poetry and literature – often by resorting to magic, mischief and cunning.

His ability to stay one step ahead of the game by anticipating change and adapting to it before anyone, god or mortal, suspected that change was even in the air was highly rated by the ancient Greeks. It has become a still more desirable attribute in today's society where change has become the only constant.

Those who possess it and capitalise upon it are recognisable by their willingness to push boundaries or break through established frontiers from which they profit hugely in terms of fame, fortune and controversy. Madonna, Michael Jackson and David Bowie who have managed to read the notoriously mercurial[13] pop music industry, and have transformed and re-invented themselves in order to remain at the forefront, are the ultimate examples of The Constant Chameleons archetype. Their motto: 'To boldly go where no man has gone before.'[14]

Dionysus' domain, like that of Hermes, is the shifting

world of reality that includes endless transformations. As the god of wine, he symbolised ecstasy and liberation on the one hand, and terror and madness on the other.

Known also as the 'loosener,' he was the embodiment of the wild, dangerous and primordial aspects of the human psyche and as such evoked more fear and fascination than the rest of the Olympian deity put together.

One can understand the particular appeal he held for the traditionally confined and, no doubt, terminally bored housewives of ancient Greece.

Intoxicated by a break in their routine, they were, according to the myths, transformed into frenzied dancers, 'girding themselves with snakes and giving suck to fawns and wolf cubs as if they were infants at the breast.' Released from domestic repression, they were invincible. 'Fire does not burn them. No weapon of iron can wound them. Fierce bulls fall to the ground, victims to numberless, tearing, female hands.'[15]

Time, however, has not diminished the female fascination for the Dionysian archetype. How else can one explain the appeal of every rebellious rock 'n' roller epitomised by the young Mick Jagger? Or Jack Nicholson who has managed to become a sex symbol and star from playing menacing, deranged danger men, not to mention the occasional werewolf? If one side of the Dionysian coin denotes horror and madness, the other symbolises freedom, comfort and bliss in abundance as demonstrated by Gerard Depardieu on screen, in the shape of his full bodied male persona, crystallised in the movie *The Green Card*. It is evident also in his private life where he makes no secret of his passion for his extensive vineyard. While

Depardieu and Nicholson are the opposite extremes of this archetype, there are several Hollywood actors who belong in the Snake Charmers category because of their hypnotic ability to attract and repel at the same time. Sometimes the charm barely disguises the menace as with John Malkovich and Gary Oldman. But often the menace is latent and, as Richard Gere, Sean Connery and Clint Eastwood prove, the threat of it being unleashed is far more compelling than its actual manifestation.

The Snake Charmers motto: 'Take a walk on the wild side.'

Dionysus also embodies dance as an elemental expression often aligned with eroticism and ecstasy. Thus all the great movers, Gene Kelly, Elvis, John Travolta, Patrick Swayze and Nureyev come under his domain. Snake Hip Seducers are not confined, however, to the dance world. Richard Gere is one. And the young Clint Eastwood is described as moving like a panther with grace.

The Snake Hip Seducers motto is: 'Float like a butterfly, sting like a bee.'

Helen of Troy was the ultimate sex object. The face that launched a thousand ships was the most highly-prized object of her time and as such was well worth fighting a war over. She was the reward offered to Paris by Aphrodite on condition he declared the goddess of love to be the fairest one of all by giving her the Golden Apple of Discord. This done, Paris picked up his prize who made no show of resistance at leaving her husband, the Greek King Menelaus. Indeed, as befits an object, Helen's role throughout was entirely passive. But make no mistake, her impact was as devastating and memorable as any goddess, a legacy she has bequeathed to her descendants. The Ultimate Babes, who most notably include Pamela Anderson, the global fantasy object of the early 90s. Helen of Troy's motto: Who dares, wins me

Footnotes:

1 Examples have been used hence the absence of Greta Garbo, Clark Gable, Elvis Presley, Marilyn Monroe and their desirable ilk, too numerous to mention.

2 From the Blue Dolphin videogram Sean Connery *Close Up*, produced by Louise Krakower, written and directed by Michael Tobias.

3 'Only Venus comes.' Marsilio Ficino, *The Book of Life*, trans. by Charles Boer (Spring Publications, Irving, Texas, 1979.

4 In terms of global bankability, Julia Roberts is the top woman, Sandra Bullock at no.4, and Meg Ryan, no.5 according to the second edition of the Ulmer Scale's 'Studio Hot list' February 1998

5 The gun is the symbol of the male ego so Day's mastery of it was a particularly subversive image for 1953, and a novel one for women who were more used to lines like: "You can't get a man with a gun."

6 Taken from The Ulmer Scale's "Studio Hot List" conducted February 1998.

7 Tennyson's Idylls of the King 'Gareth and Lynette' (1872) 1.117

8 From *Lavengro* (1851) by George Borrow.

9 From *Arts Erotica* by Edward Lucie-Smith.

10 taken from *Audrey, Her Real Story* by Alexander Walker published by Weidenfeld and Nicolson, London.

11 Taken from the *Homeric Hymn to Herakles* (Hercules)

12 Taken from *Youth* (1902) by Joseph Conrad.

13 The word actually comes from Hermes' Roman name Mercury to denote unpredictability.

14 *Star Trek* TV series, from 1966

15 From Walter F. Otto, *Dionysus: Myth and Cult* (Spring Publications, Dallas, Texas, 1981)

View from the Stars

In Hollywood, the genuine sex symbol is ready and willing yet unattainable and a touch passive. Marilyn Monroe was all these. For while it is perfectly acceptable to exude sex appeal and drive cinema audiences wild, it is quite another to exhibit naked ambition. Ideally, therefore, one should be discovered.

To be discovered excuses sex symbols from possessing such a potent force. It signifies a mixture of modesty, even unawareness on their part (heaven forbid that they should appear to depend on or actively exploit their sex appeal) while also making the point that their charisma is so powerful that it seduces everyone around them.

Lana Turner was one of the biggest stars of the 1940s and '50s but it is the way she was discovered that has earned her a place in Hollywood legend. She was 15 years old, having a coca-cola at the corner cafe across from her school, Hollywood High, when she was spotted by the owner of The Hollywood Reporter.

"Billy Wilkerson walked over to me, presented his business card. 'How do you do?' he said. 'What's your name?' I blushed. 'Judy Turner.'

"Then Billy articulated those few magical words that have become so cliché over the years: 'How would you like to be in pictures?' I looked at him, and replied, in a very sophisticated manner: 'I'll have to ask my mother!'

"Over the years, those words have been attributed to others. The magazines have had me being discovered on a stool at Schwab's Drugstore, or by God knows how many other people. But I owe it all to Billy [...] It's so odd, the way things happen – being at the right place, at the right time, I mean."[1]

Turner's discovery in 1936 was a happy accident. It just happened. And even though such innocence was exceptionally rare then, and rarer still today, the notion that talent and sex appeal will effortlessly attract notice and success remains a seductive one.

For paradoxically, when it comes to Hollywood and show business in general it is not the much vaunted American work ethic that prevails but the pre-Thatcher, covert British attitude: Work twenty hours a day by all means, just don't show it. How else can we explain that strange phenomenon of entertainers who become 'stars overnight' or 'overnight sensations' having been in the business for five, ten, even 15 years.

While actors and actresses under 35 are far more openly aspirational than the older generation, and openly admire stars like Madonna and Cher who have made effort and striving glamorous, they still balk at publicly acknowledging their sex appeal, however much they may exploit it. To do so, even today, somehow smacks of ego, arrogance, self-knowledge and a distinct lack of class.

British publicist Max Clifford says: "A lot of hypocrisy is involved. They are quite happy when everybody else says they are sex symbols although they don't want to be caught saying it themselves. In some cases they feel they have gone past the sex symbol stage – they look around and see younger rivals coming up – and they want to be taken seriously as an actor. Or perhaps they have a lifestyle which if exposed would ruin that sex symbol image."

But the reality is that looks, body and sex appeal have always been and are the standard currency of the

Hollywood star. And this is the case more than ever, now that glamour and luxury have taken a back seat and no longer draw cinema audiences the way they used to in the 1930s, 40s and 50s.

What remains unchanged is that so many stars renowned for their sex appeal come from poor or nomadic or emotionally deprived backgrounds, and have risen up-by-the-boot-straps method, capitalising on the resources they had available, namely their physical attributes and sexual chemistry. Becoming a sex symbol was the ticket out and means of achieving stardom for Sean Connery, Steve McQueen, Ava Gardner, Marilyn Monroe, Sophia Loren and Demi Moore and legions of others, past and present.

To be economically dependent on one's sex appeal, however, leaves one vulnerable, even in the case of legendary stars. Paul Newman encapsulated the precariousness of the position when he confessed to a recurring nightmare: "That on my tombstone they would write, 'Here lies Paul Newman... A great actor until one day his eyes turned brown.'"

Adding to this insecurity is that it is possible to get work as an actor without any formal training – unheard of in any other area of arts entertainment (save pop music). At the age of 20, Susan Sarandon accompanied her first husband, an actor, to an audition and was asked to read opposite him. Despite having no acting experience, she was spotted by an agent who submitted her for a film called *Joe* where she was asked to do an improvisation.

"I had no idea what that was but they explained it to me. I did it, and got the role on the spot. From that point on I kept getting the things I went up for. I have never taken an acting class. I've never studied. I just kept working and learned on the job. But because I fell into it, I never identified myself as being an actress for the first ten years."

So while stars may deploy an air of nonchalance when questioned about their sex symbol status, in most cases the nonchalance is affected. They have too much riding on it.

It is impossible to imagine Demi Moore being quoted in the News of the World newspaper, as Sigourney Weaver once was: 'I wanted to be a slut more than anything else in the world. I seriously considered making a no-holds-barred, hard-core sex movie.'

But then Weaver can afford to be humorous. Coming from a privileged family, well connected to the arts and media, and educated at Stanford University and Yale Drama School, she is able to view her sex appeal as a useful asset, one resource among many.

Her casual attitude is genuine. "I'll take my clothes off at a moment's notice," she says, referring to Hurly Burly, a Broadway play in which she stripped off for her lover, played by William Hurt. "Someone said to me that the nudity in the play was gratuitous and I replied that it probably is. Because it was optional, it was fun to do.

"If the part had depended upon taking my clothes off it would have been an issue. As it is, I think it's funny – the contrast between the lovers' earnest conversation and the frivolity of ripping off each other's clothes. Quite honestly, I think nude scenes are fine. I've yet to do a film where nudity was anything more than distracting."

Most of Weaver's contemporaries, however, are not in the same boat as she is the first to point out. "Most actresses in my category are being sent a lot of scripts that are old, clunky versions of women taking off their clothes. Only now they are playing successful business women and that's supposed to make it acceptable. So boring.

" It's a pleasure to turn down these parts as a bigger name because I think people used to think 'well, she's this smart Alec from Yale.' The thing is that somebody very good will probably end up doing this kind of role.

"It's not as if I am puritanical. But there's something about the violence and the sex... Just selfishly I can't imagine spending three months of my life on a film set discussing what to take off, when and how much humiliation I should go through before I experience some great awakening of who I am. I think it's absurd. Who cares? Why watch for two hours while a woman works out with some sadistic lover? Send the woman to a psychiatrist."

Which brings us to the vexed question of whether or not sex symbols are particularly susceptible to being exploited by the Hollywood industry. The legendary actress Joan Crawford who was a sex symbol in the 1930s, discussed this with film academic Jeanine Basinger, saying: "When I was coming through in the 1920s, during the transition from silent films to sound, there were very few of us in the business who had anything. We came mostly from poverty. The studio worked us very hard. They had enormous control over our lives. But we had careers. We had money – things we never would have had otherwise. Most of us never thought of it as exploitation because we were paid for the work we wanted to do and we knew it was a business." Basinger believes this remains an accurate assessment of the sex symbol situation.

But Crawford was a hard-headed woman, one of Hollywood's greatest survivors. In contrast, many sex symbols are noted for their emotional fragility, often borne out of unstable early lives.

Marilyn Monroe was not the first and will not be the last star who hoped to find in Hollywood what she couldn't find in her childhood. "I wanted more than anything to be loved. Love to me then and now means being wanted. It seemed nobody wanted me... I was nine years old when I entered the orphanage and eleven when Aunt Grace finally took me out."[2]

Dudley Moore, at the height of his fame, confided that he was embarrassed at how publicly and interminably he talked about love being the important element in his life and yet found it virtually impossible to maintain long-term relationships. Clearly, he adored the affection, attention and adulation of the public but responding to this general love was so time consuming, it left him little time to develop and sustain personal love.

"I express myself principally through love for people, for lovers and friends," he said. "My pleasures, really, are with people and my work."

Moore's professionalism and consideration in his dealings with media are legendary. He is the only international star I know who regularly returned journalists' phone calls and letters personally despite the overwhelming demands on his time and attention. He would always say it was because he liked to be in control and did not like delegating matters. "I like to make my own decisions on things apart from anything else... The terrible thing is that sometimes I have to get my secretary to phone back my friends to say that I've had their call and I'll phone them back as soon as possible."

But when probed further he admitted that he had a deep-seated fear of disappointing anyone, for he craved approval and wanted the world and his brother to love him as if somehow they could make up for what he found lacking in his childhood.

Dudley Moore would no doubt agree with James Dean who once said: "One of the deepest drives of human nature is the desire to be appreciated, the longing to be liked, to be held in esteem, to be a sought-after person... There are six needs in life: love, security, self-esteem, recognition, new experiences, and last, but not least, the need for creative expression."

Sex symbols' early lives may spur them on to make good in Hollywood but leave them ill-equipped to handle the pressures. The irony is that to survive and thrive in a dream factory, one has to have a very firm grip on professional reality.

Photojournalist George Barris, with whom Marilyn Monroe collaborated on a book about her life, observed: "I could see that Marilyn was a dreamer, too. She had been taken advantage of so often that she found comfort in the make-believe parts she grew up to portray on the screen. When she completed a film she could discard the character she had played and go on to another for a while, but her real life was impossible to discard. She wanted to make her past disappear, but she knew it would always return to haunt her."

A solid marriage and family life are invariably given as a star's best defence against burn out, addiction and tragedy. But this has always eluded the majority of the Hollywood élite, especially when they marry each other and one or both happen to be sex symbols. As Mel Gibson said: "This is the most licentious and tempting city in the world – and in this business it is easy to fall prey and be seduced by it."

So much so, that an enduring celebrity partnership is regarded as news. Paul Newman's response to how he avoided the temptation of affairs has never been bettered: "Why should you fool around with a hamburger when you have steak at home?"

His wife, Joanne Woodward says: "My great grand-mother said, 'Don't marry anybody unless you can imagine talking over the breakfast table for 50 years.' Now that makes enormous sense if you actually think about it because the sex and all that may go away but you sure as hell have got to have breakfast.

"There is nobody in my life that I can imagine talking and listening to for over 50 years except my husband, with the possible exception of one of my closest friends who happens to be male. We chat away all the time."

Woodward may be a brilliant Oscar winning actress in her own right but in common with most stars' wives she has been the one to make the concessions necessary for the marriage to succeed, as Newman publicly acknowledged. "Joanne really gave up her career for me, to help me raise my children, to stick by me and make the marriage work."

"Sure, it's true," says Woodward. "But no-one puts a gun to your head and says have children. My generation did it because that was what people said we should do. I didn't know anything about children, I didn't particularly like children. Then I got married and said, 'oh well, now I have to have children.' Idiotic isn't it?

"Sometimes I look back and think, 'what a shame.' I have three lovely daughters and really didn't spend enough time with them when they were children, and then worried about the time I did spend with them. If only I had been able to say sensibly and in a mature fashion, 'This is what I really want.'

"I have told my children, 'My darlings, I love you all. I adore you. I suppose it would have made more sense if I hadn't had you all because I did spend a lot of time moaning and groaning and bitching about the effect of children on my career. But it was my choice.

"I know actresses to whom motherhood should never have happened because they care about their careers to such an extreme. Also, the difficulty even nowadays is that most women still haven't gotten to the point of being able to say it's alright not to have children."

A pregnant sex symbol is a contradiction in terms, judging by the general Hollywood view and to be fair, one shared by the movie-going public. For although a sex symbol is at some subconscious level expected to exude the promise of fertility, concrete proof of her fruitfulness is deemed to detract from her sex appeal.

Actress Demi Moore highlighted this paradox when she broke with convention by refusing to go quietly and reappearing after the birth. Instead, she broadcast her pregnant bulge on the cover of Vanity Fair magazine. The photographs shocked at the time and are still remembered today which is an indication of just how deeply rooted the sex symbol stereotype is embedded in our psyche.

Indeed, Moore is a high profile example of the modern woman striving to 'have it all'. "She has children whom she adores, a career and is married to someone who is incredibly demanding," says agent Lindy King. "And she is trying to juggle it all against inscrutable odds. Yes, she does have nannies and assistants and trainers but she works hard at keeping it altogether. I feel, give her a break. This is a woman who has absolutely made it happen for herself."

She is also subject to the pressures of being married to a fellow star and sex symbol, Bruce Willis. Their much-publicised, and often turbulent, relationship is probably not helped by the notorious perk of Hollywood stardom – the sheer abundance of beautiful, young, available women.

The difference between top male stars and their female counterparts says King, is that the women are still expected to be little homemakers and thus the balance is out of kilter. "The man is the hunter-gatherer and at the end of the day he doesn't like the role reversal, and the woman is left on her own. So she gets involved in a series of less and less sustaining relationships.

"Men aren't nurturers or carers, and while they may do it in the first flush of love or infatuation, they are not going to keep the home fires burning day after day, month after month, year after year."

Of course, there has always been the phenomenon of caretaker husbands – wealthy men, usually older than their star wives, with careers far removed from show business.

But more often than not actors and actresses fall for each other. At star level it is generally a case of charisma attracting charisma. Tom Cruise and Nicole Kidman are a case in point. Their combined charismatic image as the beautiful, classy celebrity couple rivals their individual sexy on-screen personas.

But when it comes to sizzling sexual chemistry no one comes close to Bogart and Bacall, undoubtedly the iconic Hollywood couple. Their status was sealed with Lauren Bacall's first kiss in her first movie in 1943, *To Have and Have Not*. She clearly electrified Humphrey Bogart when she took the initiative and kissed him, and then swaggered seductively to the door to impart that famous line, "If you want me, just whistle. You know how to whistle don't you? Just put your lips together and blow."

Actors and actresses are commonly drawn to each other because of a high-voltage attraction that develops from working together intensively on a film set (usually short-lived). Actress Grace Kelly, at one point labelled 'Miss Home breaker' by L.A. Confidential magazine, was notorious for her affairs with her leading men, numbering among her conquests William Holden who for a short time left his wife for her.

Chemistry apart, the reason most often given for celebrity coupling is that being in the same profession they understand the pressures both are under.

Actor Eric Stoltz whose partner is Bridget Fonda, says:

"I live with an actress and in the past dated one. I feel I know them. Being in the same profession doesn't make the relationship harder. At least, it doesn't in this one. I don't feel there's any competition. We have discussed this. She really wants to work and work and her different approach makes me question my own. I am not that career-oriented. And I have been involved with women who are a little bit scared by that and who are more driven than I am.

"Once I was in a relationship with an actress who was disturbed that I was not driven to be the most successful person around. I felt that was a sexist attitude and I very much resented her attitude which is probably why we did not stay together."

Even where the competitive element is absent from the relationship there remains the strain of working apart from each other for months on end. "I might do a play in New York. She might be making a film elsewhere," says Stoltz. "It is a question of logistics and priorities. Somehow, we have to find the time to have a life together."

But it is fame, supposedly the great reward Hollywood can confer upon a star, which poses the greatest threat to long-lasting relationships. And sex symbols tend to be more famous than any other kind of star because their sex appeal fascinates the public so, and arouses an apparently insatiable desire to know everything about them.

Female stars are acknowledged to have a tougher time from the paparazzi and videorazzi because their male counterparts are more likely to hit back physically (this can backfire though – a videorazzo can earn $10,000 or more a minute showing footing of a star behaving badly).

Actress Gillian Anderson has been hounded by the British press in Vancouver, Canada where *The X-Files* TV series is filmed. On two occasions, they barged into her trailer and refused to leave until they got the photographs of her they wanted.

"You already feel vulnerable because the nature of the work demands that you expose parts of yourself and so you feel more vulnerable than say a famous writer or painter. I have now developed a shield of protection around me. I can usually spot paparazzi a mile away and see cameras out of the corners of my eyes.

"The underlying problem is that although we complain about the paparazzi, and justifiably so, they and the newspapers make money from us because people want that information. So it's the fans, the people partly responsible for our livelihood who are also partly responsible for the intensity of the attention.

"I don't wish I hadn't experienced fame. What bothers me is that because we have decided to be public figures the press and paparazzi feel they have a right to intricate, intimate details about our lives."

The truth is that the screen persona has never been enough for the audience. During the studio days, Hollywood brazenly manufactured fictional lives and loves for its stars. Today, the press promises the real thing and in the eyes of its chosen celebrity prey have metamorphosed into some kind of pit bull media monster intent upon assaulting, eroding and finally destroying their privacy.

Actress Susan Sarandon's relationship with actor Tim

Robbins, 12 years younger than her, and by whom she had a baby at the age of 45, was a tabloid press dream come true.

"It is hard when people want to know about very personal issues, when you open a newspaper and read about what's happening in your life. I turned down a job because I knew I was pregnant. It was so early I hadn't even been to the doctor but it was made public. That, I felt, was a real violation and I felt betrayed. Things like that happen. You find out that your boyfriend has been going out with someone else and it becomes melodramatic.

"But anybody who says fame bothers them is completely full of shit. You can't be in this business and not want anyone to see you. That's a complete contradiction in terms. Of course you don't want to receive weird letters or have people sit down next to you while you are having dinner in a restaurant. You don't want people to threaten the life of your child or to feel your child is in jeopardy because she's recognisable. And there are times you don't feel like signing an autograph.

"But the people who usually approach me have something very specific to say and although there are some who shout and squeal at a high decibel level, you just have to accept that's part of it.

"Fame can sometimes be an advantage. I have never understood why anybody would want to know what an actress thinks but it enables me to get on TV and talk about the causes I believe in. I remember talking about Aids on a talk show at a time when Aids campaigners couldn't get time on TV for anything. I guess you have to be careful not to let it control you, though."

Mel Gibson who admits to having developed a fortress mentality in the face of overwhelming fame recalled its destructive impact during his early *Mad Max* days.

"I had a drinking career… It really was a waste of time and money and health. But you only see that in retrospect. Man, I wish I'd stopped earlier.

"I was at the beginning of the road to ruin. There are degrees of ruination but I didn't get very far before I thought there is something wrong with all this and extract-ed myself from this whole world for a year and a half."[3]

Observing the effects of fame on Gibson today, one cannot help being aware of the way in which his image has expanded to cover the globe and swallowed up his personal space in the process. Here is a man who in mate-rial terms has the world at his feet and yet in an innate personal sense has less access to it than the average private citizen.

'I can't go to many places, this sounds funny, where I am accepted in a normal fashion. By that I mean it's hard to find a place where they are relaxed with your pres-ence.'[4] The private Gibson is bound by fame to a handful of exclusive refuges, one of which being a celebrity members-only club where he can indulge in the occasion-al Havana cigar. But there are the fortunate few who appear thoroughly comfortable with their image, regard-ing it as an exaggerated extension of themselves. Jack Nicholson and Arnold Schwarzenegger are typical of this rare breed. They are movie stars first, actors second.

"There are actors, and there are actors who are celebri-ties and stars. As a star you carry a lot of baggage with you which means people know a lot about you, about your background, your private life and this affects people's perceptions of you and makes you less believable in certain roles," says Schwarzenegger.

"That's why guys like Marlon Brando and Robert De Niro shy away from the media because they don't want anyone to know the real them. It enables them to play an enormous range of characters. I have to approach it differently but I've never found it a drawback because I like the characters I have chosen to play."

Struggling to reconcile the image with their humanity is the norm, however, as the roll call of illustrious male and female sex symbols railing against their predicament (ever since the invention of the Hollywood vamp in the 1920s) bears out.

At the root of their dilemma is the discrepancy between their physical endowments which just are, and their potential. Robert Redford was speaking for many a sex symbol when he said: 'All my life I've been dogged by guilt because I feel there is this difference between the way I look and what I feel inside. I suppose I look all right but I can never figure what that's got to do with talent, or virtue, or anything. Besides, it's extremely dangerous to take anybody at face value.'

The degree to which the public view is at variance from how stars personally perceive themselves adds to their unease. Actresses Jamie Lee Curtis and Gillian Anderson have experimented with developing sexy images of themselves to show audiences and the industry that there is this other side to them and so avoid being pigeon-holed professionally.

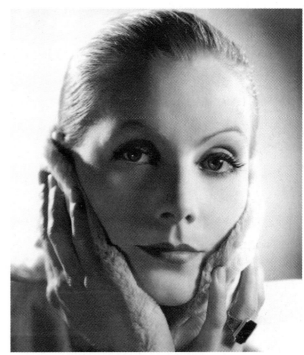

The divine and heavenly face of Aphrodite - Greta Garbo.

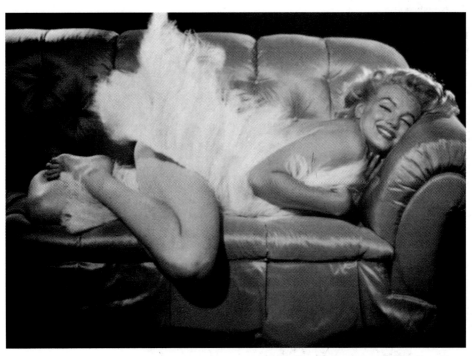

Marilyn Monroe in her heyday.

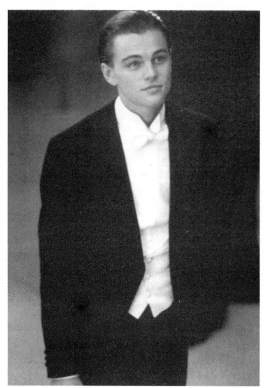

Leonardo DiCaprio - Adonis incarnate.

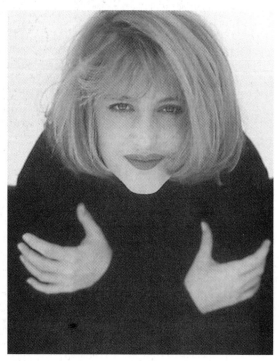

Gillian Anderson - without Scully's overcoat.

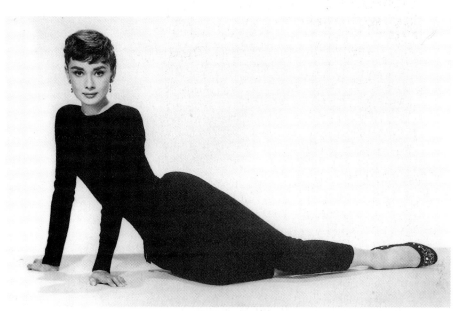

Audrey Hepburn - Air Diva of the 1960s.

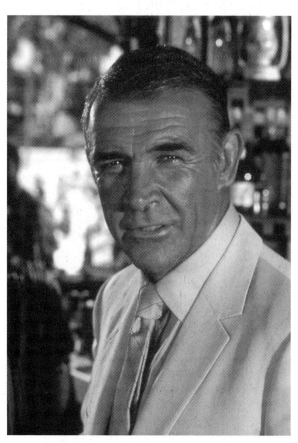

Sean Connery - the 'Great Unknockable'.

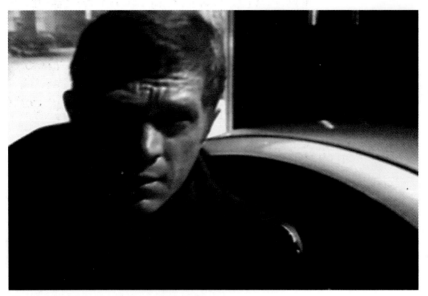

Steve McQueen with a Puma.

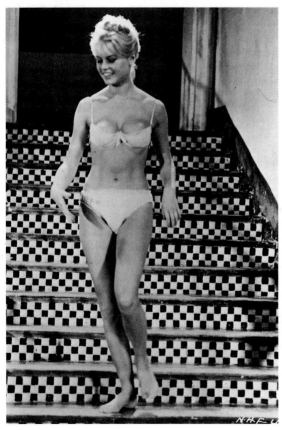

Brigitte Bardot - the golden, glowing Aphrodite.

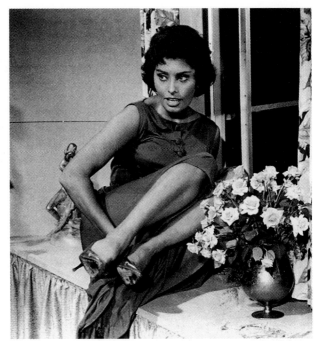

Sophia Loren - The Ultimate Diva.

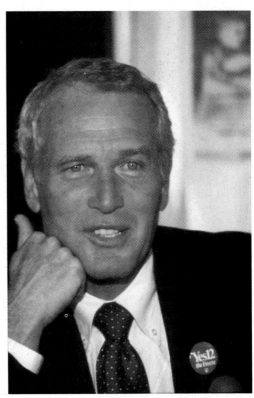

Paul Newman - a Rebel and a Rogue.

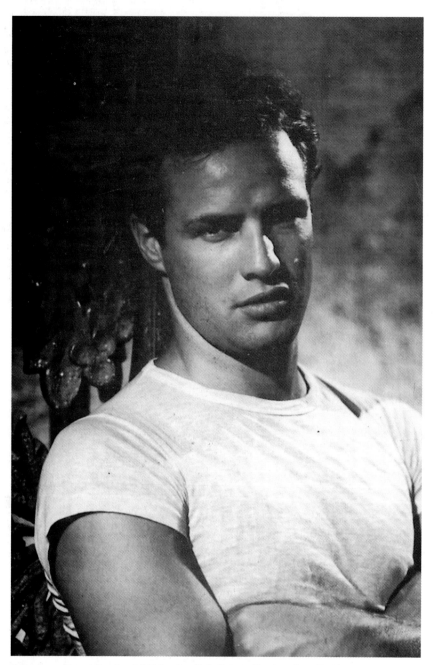

Marlon Brando in 1951; youthful Apollo in the flesh.

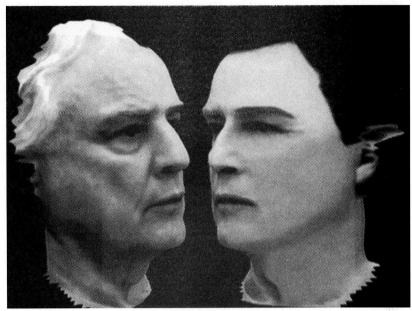

Stripping away the years - age morph geometry in action.

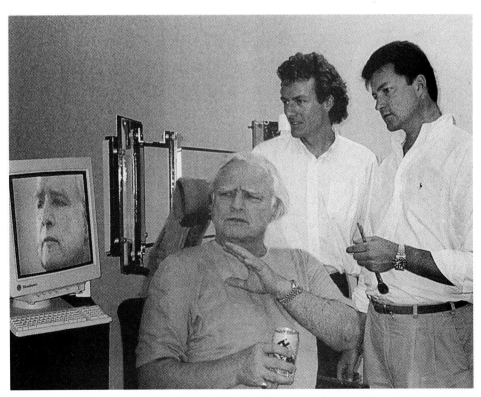

Marlon Brando examining computer scans of his mannerisms.

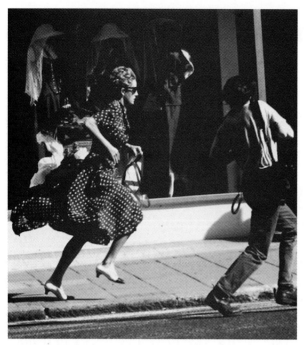

Diana, Princess of Wales. Sex symbols often have a price to pay for their popularity.

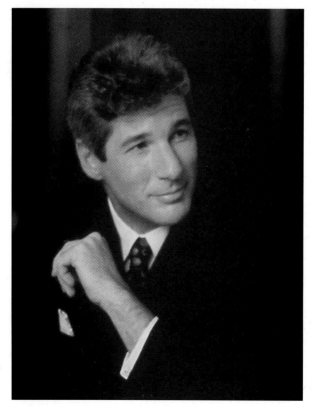

Richard Gere - Snake Charmer.

Curtis once had a dream in which she was photographed standing at a bend in the road next to a sign warning, 'Danger, curves ahead.' She had the sign painted and posed beside it, her own curves prominently revealed.

Anderson agreed to do a couple of deliberately sexy and suggestive magazine covers. A slew of others, whilst not intentionally sexy, emerged as such.

Thus, despite having found fame in genres not normally associated with eroticism and sex appeal – horror movies and comedies (Curtis) and sci-fi (Anderson) – they are publicly acknowledged as sex symbols.

"I still don't know what I feel about being a sex symbol," says Anderson. "It's flattering but I'm not sure where it fits in. It's not who I am when I am changing my daughter's diapers or when I am walking around in my casual clothes. In fact, people are surprised to see how normal I am, how normally I dress."

Curtis has a similar take on the subject. "I think it's great that men perceive me as a sex symbol. I'm flattered. But the minute I start thinking of myself as one, I'll stop being one. I was a tomboy, I still am. I was never what I call a slut-girl sex symbol. I don't wear slut clothes – often. Once in a while I'll throw on something just to liven things up but that's no indication of the real me. It's interesting watching the reaction of people who have seen me in a film and then meet me. They look at me and say, 'But you don't look anything like…'"

If a consequence of mass sex appeal is fame, the reverse is also true. Graham Greene's observation that fame is a powerful aphrodisiac is supported by this wry story related to me by singer-songwriter Barry Manilow.

"My grandmother said to me, 'Barry, you were always a clever boy and I knew you would be a success. You were always talented, and I knew you'd be famous. But how you got to be sexy and good-looking, I'll never understand."

Modern day stars have also to contend with completely false photographic images of themselves, resulting from the rapid growth of digital imaging. Where before their photographic image was a fixed entity, it is now fluid and oh-so-easy to manipulate. It can be mass-produced, switched on or off, expanded, put on hold, and fed into the Internet where it can be dissected, then transposed on to strange bodies and photographed in still stranger pornographic poses.

"It's gone crazy," says Dennis Davidson of DDA, an international entertainment public relations company. "On the Internet I came across a German programme showing pornographic pictures of Antonio Banderas. They mixed and matched his face with an anonymous someone posing naked on the Net. If they had a naked picture of Banderas that would be bad enough but creating this stuff is unbelievable."

Oddly, Gillian Anderson, who has more than 2,700,000 references on the Web devoted to her, dismisses such abuses.

"Yes, my head has been placed on other people's bodies and no, there isn't anything legal you can do about it. But to tell you the truth it doesn't bother me. It's not hurting anybody. It's not hurting me. I'd be much more concerned if they were actually real naked pictures taken of me when I was younger that I had forgotten about."

Fake or provocative photographs are one thing but words are quite another matter. Anderson's mother may have been "a little taken aback" by the overall sexy image but she, like her daughter, was far more concerned about the slant of the accompanying interview. "The articles that are written about me are building up an image that isn't true. That's what I find really disturbing. For this reason and for the sake of privacy I have been very vague in many interviews about myself, my childhood, my family and my relationships – and I have, especially over the past couple of years, kept my private life very close to my chest."

The experiences of actresses Glenn Close and Isabella Rossellini illustrate the positive and negative aspects of a sexy image.

Until the1987 film *Fatal Attraction,* Glenn Close was predominantly seen as a good actress with a nice line in repressed/icy women and warm housewives/mothers. By playing the modern version of the sado-masochistic vamp – the independent woman who is deadly, however, she developed a sexy aura and box office clout.

Michael Douglas says: "I remember telling her, 'look, you are known as a good actress but because of this sexy, romantic role another side of you is blossoming.' Guys were calling me, saying, 'I always liked her as an actress but now I really fancy her.' So I advised her to capitalise on her new image."

Close managed to strike the happy balance that is the envy of most stars – she was perceived as a dynamite actress who could act sexy and was consequently credited with sex appeal. She avoided the sex symbol tag because it was what she was able to portray that increased her Hollywood stature, not what she intrinsically is.

Actress Isabella Rossellini's beauty – at 30 she landed a Lancôme modelling contract worth $2 million – and her heritage as Ingrid Bergman's daughter, have conspired to make her a glamorous sex symbol.

Her decision to play the masochistic Dorothy in the 1986 film *Blue Velvet* proved highly controversial owing to her public image. On one hand, the director David Lynch was lambasted for exploiting her sexiness and on the other, he was accused of destroying the looks of a beautiful woman.

Rossellini recalls: "I was devastated that they thought I was trying to be sexy. Dorothy had been raped physically and mentally by her son's kidnapper – if there was one thing she wasn't, it was sexy. But because I was filmed naked, I was accused of trying to be sexy.

"Then it was said that David took me and spoiled me by deliberately making me ugly. They said I was fat. Well, it was important that my character wasn't thin, healthy and athletic. I mean this was a film about the horror of rape and kidnap, and I was playing a woman who had been completely degraded.

Three years after completing *Blue Velvet* she admitted to having seen it only once because she says, "I was so hurt by the reaction. Instead of watching the film and giving it the attention it really deserved, I would be replaying in my head all the comments about how fat I am, or thinking, 'here's the part where they say David destroyed me.'"

What got Rossellini into trouble is that she is a sex symbol, a model one at that, and the image she portrayed in *Blue Velvet* flew in the face of the sophisticated European glamour she has come to epitomise – hence the furore.

Black sex symbols are in a particularly invidious position. While their box office clout depends on appealing to as wide an audience as possible, they are expected to adhere to some hard and fast rules when going global. If they are perceived as going 'too far,' the black community especially the women may see it as a betrayal.

For successful black movie actors are also role models and therefore it is deemed fitting that their sex appeal be deployed in politically correct circumstances.

Elsie B. Washington, a former Editor of the US black magazine Essence, says: "I remember one movie where a white woman makes a seductive appeal to Denzel Washington and he turns her down. There was a collective sigh of relief from all the black women in the audience because in reality so many black men are with white women. It partly explains why we tend to favour black stars although, of course, there are white sex symbols who have some appeal for black women.

"Even though Denzel is regarded as a sex symbol among white women, he makes a point of not having kissing scenes or sex with white women in his movies. It is important because he is someone we look up to and admire as a hero. He is a symbol of righteousness we would say and we want him to do right and be right. He is like the John Wayne of the black race.

"His appeal is not down to just his looks or professional code of behaviour. It has to do with his whole persona. He's married. He is faithful to his wife. He treats his family well. He's taken them all to Africa on safari. He does charitable works and gives money to good causes."

In contrast, she dismisses Sidney Poitier as a whites-only sex symbol and Diana Ross an "unreal fantasy figure." Today's black sex symbols are listed as actors Will Smith and Wesley Snipes, Tina Turner, Whitney Houston and TV actress Halle Berry. But Denzel Washington aside, the ultimate black icons are retired athletes: basketball player Michael Jordan and boxer Muhammad Ali.

The Hollywood star is a conduit, an interactive force whose two-dimensional image can somehow communicate in 3-D and arouse 3-D responses from the audience in return. By their very nature then, star sex symbols are among the most potent communicators of all, hence their huge box office appeal.

Film academic Jeanine Basinger writes: "A movie star may or may not be able to act by theatrical standards, but he or she must be able to create a relationship with viewers. That is the secret of stardom..."[5]

As Hollywood is all about image on and off screen, good looks are what the industry takes as its starting point. For as pioneering sexologist Havelock Ellis pointed out in 1918 in his Studies in the Psychology of Sex: "Practically speaking, so far as man and his immediate ancestors are concerned, the sexual and extra-sexual factors of beauty have been interwoven from the first... It is not surprising, therefore, that from the point of view of sexual selection, vision should be the supreme sense and that the love-thoughts of men have always been a perpetual meditation of beauty."

Thus the power of the camera in detecting, illuminating, and some would controversially say even creating, an aura of sex appeal has long been acknowledged by Hollywood.

While the essence of sex appeal is always tantalisingly indefinable, we know it instantly when we see it – and feel it. To my mind, the best description of an authentic star sex symbol comes from director Rouben Mamoulian about Greta Garbo whom he directed in the 1933 film *Queen Christina*.

"What made Greta unique? First, it was her look. She had the ideal photogenic face. Before we started shooting Christina, I made some tests so that I would know how to light her properly. When we looked at the finished film, I thought, 'Am I crazy, or is it possible that whatever we use she looks beautiful?' I challenged her cameraman Billy Daniels: 'Let's see if we can ruin her.' So he took a light and put it below her face, in the harshest kind of grotesque angle. She still looked magnificent. It was a God-given gift Greta had, as opposed to, say, Dietrich. Marlene looked beautiful on film, but it sometimes took two hours to light her.

"Second, Garbo was thoroughly intuitive. Her subconscious has sensitivities to moods, to subtleties of emotion and feeling that cannot be reasonably explained. With Garbo, there was no point in being logical. Instead, I used metaphors. For instance, once I said: 'Greta, you know the way a flower opens to the light? That's the way your face will look when you see John (her co-star). From those few words, she knew instinctively what I meant – and gave it to me. It was one subconscious talking to another.

"Third, Garbo had grace of movement, which can make or break a performer. She moved beautifully. But in her case, there was an added element which was something of a mystery. It was her capacity for stirring up the spectator's imagination. With certain actors, they call it charisma... charm.

"Some people can walk into a room, you look at them, and there is nothing there. Someone else walks in, and you can't take your eyes off of her, or him. There's always something there. With Garbo there was always more in the spectator's eye and mind than there was on screen."[6]

Actress Virginia McKenna, who worked with Gary Cooper in *The Wreck of the Mary Deare*, recalls: "I did this cameo role because I so wanted to work with him. Gary Cooper's charisma wasn't just something that emerged on the screen. It came from within. It was there when I was working with him, actually it was always present. I remember being at a drinks party and he was so compelling that all of us were drawn to him, acutely aware of him yet at the same time trying not to look. You could feel him."

I witnessed Muhammad Ali exercise the same magnetic pull in the late 1970s as he walked through a restaurant in the London Hilton Hotel. Diners with their back to him felt him first and then involuntarily turned to stare, awestruck with pleasure. He moved with unparalleled power and liquid grace, and we knew we were watching the fittest, finest looking and physically perfect man we were likely to see in all our lifetimes. Reputation did not come into it. Had he not been the most famous boxer in the world, he still would have stopped traffic – Muhammad Ali was the business.

Doyen of film publicists, Paramount's Leslie Pound, who worked on the 1953 Hollywood film *Roman Holiday*, considers its stars Audrey Hepburn and Gregory Peck peerless. Of all the actors and actresses he has worked with through the years – and they include father and son Kirk and Michael Douglas, Tom Cruise and Harrison Ford – Hepburn gets his vote for possessing the most charisma.

But it is Sophia Loren, he recalls, who gave an unforgettable demonstration of just how mesmerising the combined aura of stardom and sex appeal can be.

"We were on an international tour together where she was promoting her book and a Michael Winner movie, Firepower. I remember following Sophia as she entered through the main doors of the Imperial Hotel in Tokyo into a lobby the size of a football field. She never went through side doors, it was always centre stage for Sophia, and almost instinctively I felt I had to fall dutifully two steps behind her.

"She had this swing bag which swung as she undulated naturally through the lobby. I swear there wasn't an eye that wasn't drawn towards her in that vast space. It was uncanny. So much so that when we got upstairs I said, 'I can't believe the attention you can cause just by walking through a lobby.' She laughed and said, 'I am Sophia.' And I thought well, that's it."

It is what Baz Bamigboye, the British Daily Mail's chief show business correspondent describes as an "incredible force-field of sex."

"Connery has it," he says, recalling the time the modern-day Zeus stepped out of a cab and held the door open for Bamigboye's wife. "She didn't know who it was at first but she felt physically compelled to turn and look at him. I thought she was going to walk off with him such was his magnetic impact."

Sharon Stone is another star who has it, he says, and is able to turn it on by sheer willpower. "At one Cannes Film Festival both the weather and news were dull. Sharon who was publicising some deal was wearing this wonderful dress with a very full skirt. The photographer asked her to turn round and as she swirled round the effect was electric. We could feel this extraordinary charge, and the camera caught it."

The real test of who has and who hasn't got sex appeal in the flesh, he believes, is when the stars emerge from their limousines and ascend the red carpeted Palais steps at the Cannes Film Festival, flanked on both sides by hundreds of paparazzi and camera crews.

"There are the people you see going up and there are those you don't see because they just haven't got it. It's a great star indicator to me. Gerard Depardieu, Terence Stamp, Sigourney Weaver, Jamie Lee Curtis and Kim Basinger have it. Age has nothing to do with it. Claudia Cardinale and Burt Lancaster have it.

"But Val Kilmer doesn't have it; neither does Chris O'Donnell, he was wooden as a board. And you wouldn't necessarily look twice at Warren Beatty going up those stairs, even though he comes across on screen."

Beatty, who was a huge sex symbol because of the movies *Bonnie and Clyde*, and *Splendor in the Grass* in which he made Hollywood history by French kissing on screen, belongs to that breed of star who has innate sex appeal. But these days, at least, he seems content to keep it sheathed, reserving his homme fatale attraction for the screen.

This ability to turn sex appeal on and off like an electric light has frequently been observed by publicists, agents and journalists alike. I remember a 1987 interview with Michael Douglas in New York. He was discussing how his long-time intention to turn a particular book that explored the dynamics of lust and sexual chemistry into a screenplay had been pre-empted by the *Fatal Attraction* project. He paused to pour a glass of water and as he turned it was as if an internal switch went on and he quite literally radiated sexual magnetism. It was dazzling and totally undiscriminating – I felt like a rabbit caught in car headlights – and taking the coward's way out I changed the subject to his family.

Publicist Patric Scott who worked on promoting *Fatal Attraction*, says: "All the women representatives from the magazines went bananas over Michael Douglas. He was their fantasy. I think Douglas definitely has a very physical presence. He is very easy with himself – you have to remember that as a child of the industry his image is not radically different from who he is. Obviously in his private life he is a sensual man and feels that this is all part and parcel of himself and you see it reflected in his choice of roles.

"Most stars, however, turn on their public persona. I see it. When handling their interviews you are dealing with them from the moment you meet them until you wave them off at the airport, and most of them are very distant because they want to guard their image. That's why when someone comes in for several days to do interviews you nearly always find they say the same thing.

"You notice the difference looking after British and American stars. It's not that the British are more professional, it's that they just get on with it whereas the Americans seem to inhabit this image. Before they go out anywhere there is this whole performance of re-inhabiting their persona.

"It irks me that US publicists work so much on the image that it almost takes on a life of its own. Very often when you eventually meet the star you are surprised at how much you like him or her because the American publicist's image, this fictional other person, is so different from the actor or actress you are looking after."

Many stars, according to those who work alongside them, are so intent upon creating and maintaining their professional image that they lose sight of their roots, terra firma, and ultimately themselves.

"You don't meet many stars who are realistic and I've met a lot of them in 30 years. Paul Newman is one of the few. Nor do you find that they are married to someone who is level-headed like Joanne Woodward," says publicist Max Clifford.

Patric Scott concurs: "Sean Connery is a rare mix. He is gruff but warm, slightly distant, very aware of who he is but someone who has never forgotten his roots. Some actors are so image conscious you wonder whether they ever drop the façade, even when they get home. They certainly don't remember their roots."

To be fair, if a star is going to stay at the top these days, savvy marketing of one's image is as important as an astute choice of roles. The élite tends to favour the '15 minute' school of publicity exposure, whereby they make themselves available in measured amounts.

Sean Connery, Harrison Ford and Tom Cruise are past masters of the minimalist interview. They deliver just enough superbly well to keep media and audiences hooked and wanting more until their next promotional appearance. And it works. It stretches out their shelf life, avoids over-exposure and adds to their aura of unattainability.

Ford and Cruise, whose 'yes' and 'no' answers at the start of their careers were a journalist's worst nightmare, have with maturity become what is known in the trade as 'good interviews' and, if inclined, are able to carry on an interview as though it were a conversation.

They are at their best, however, communicating with their audiences. When Cruise was promoting *Mission Impossible* in Germany he felt he had not spent enough time with the fans outside the theatre where the film was being premiered. "So he went back out and really worked the crowd," recalls the film's publicist. "He shook hands, looked them in the eye and signed t-shirts and autographs for a further 20 minutes. Some guy said, 'Great sunglasses.' Tom replied, 'You like them?' And he took them off and gave them to him. Nice touch."

Cruise was a sex symbol to be reckoned with before he made *Top Gun*. But his dare devil sex appeal in this film, combined with the uniform, catapulted him into the super-stardom league. The same potent combination in the film *An Officer and a Gentleman* also made a superstar of Richard Gere.

It is undeniable that clothes can play as important a role in accentuating the sexiness of the wearer as no clothes at all. This is especially the case in costume dramas. Actor Sean Bean, for instance, is regarded as a sex symbol in the British TV series *Sharpe*, set in the Napoleonic Wars, in which he plays a rough diamond private who rises to Major on merit; a swashbuckling mix of outstanding bravery and heroic moral fibre. And undoubtedly his costume serves to enhance his appeal.

"His no-frills uniform shows off his great physique to its best advantage and is an indicator of his no-nonsense character. Bean wears very tight-fitting black trousers, knee-high brown boots, figure-hugging army black jacket nipped in at the waist and deeply open at the top to reveal a hint of white shirt. The only colour is a slash of red provided by his sash," says marketing consultant Carole Stewart. "The effect is devastatingly sexy and macho, particularly as the officers in the other regiments are awash with colour and look like peacocks in comparison."

But Bean's sex appeal is inextricably bound up with the role of Sharpe. He is not generally considered sexy as Agent 006 turned villain in the Bond movie *GoldenEye* or as the terrorist in *Patriot Games*.

So if we accept that one can become a sex symbol because the role is sexy – remember Colin Firth as D'Arcy in the TV adaptation of *Pride and Prejudice* – and not necessarily because of some intrinsic x-factor, then surely the likelihood of being able to manufacture one increases, doesn't it?

Contrary to myth, however, examples of completely manufactured star sex symbols are rare and successful ones still rarer. Hollywood traditionally would 'try out' innumerable young, good-looking men and women by sticking them in movies, and intelligently leave it to audiences to sift through them until they found someone they liked. Usually, it was only at this point that the film studios moved in, made that someone over – sometimes unrecognisably so – and built him or her up.

One of the most memorable exceptions, however, was the prototype blonde sex kitten, Kim Novak who was the product of an astonishing revenge gesture.

Harry Cohn, the then President of Columbia Pictures was furious with his big box office sex symbol Rita Hayworth whose career was in jeopardy owing to her controversial affair with the very much-married Prince Aly Khan and her suddenly lackadaisical approach to film commitments. Cohn swore he would create a beautiful sex goddess to take her place. Hayworth paid no heed and Kim Novak was the bombshell result

Modern-day Hollywood also occasionally tries its hand at creating a star sex symbol.

Actor Matthew McConaughey was a recent high profile attempt. He came from nowhere, according to one international publicist, to play the lead in the John Grisham movie *A Time to Kill* and made the July 1996 cover of the US Vanity Fair magazine as the next big heart-throb.

Hollywood's timing was, to put it mildly, unfortunate. McConaughey's carefully orchestrated career was soon to be eclipsed by the emergence of Leonardo DiCaprio, the hottest actor-Adonis since James Dean in the mid-1950s.

Moreover, DiCaprio was the people's spontaneous choice. Around the world, teenage girls fell in love with the romantic Bohemian character Jack in the 1998 film *Titanic* and even more deeply in love with the actor who played him.

Having in extreme cases returned to watch DiCaprio 30 or 40 times, they rented videos of his older films. The combined rentals of *Marvin's Room*, *The Basketball Diaries* and *Romeo + Juliet* increased 61 per cent in the three weeks after *Titanic* opened in British cinemas. Steep rises were also recorded in Japan and US. But perhaps the hottest video item has been *Total Eclipse* because it features DiCaprio in a full-frontal nude scene. Predictably, the film that followed *Titanic*, *The Man in the Iron Mask* which co-starred established stars Gerard Depardieu, John Malkovich and Jeremy Irons was sold and marketed on DiCaprio's name – and indisputably profited by it.

"The extraordinary thing is that in the first half of the film he plays a pig, the most obnoxious little man who ever walked this earth," says publicist Dennis Davidson. "But my daughter, who I took again to see it, didn't care. She loved it. It was Leonardo."

DiCaprio illustrates the phenomenal impact of authentic sex appeal when exposed to today's highly sophisticated and global communications network. At the same time, the proliferation and intrusiveness of the media has made it much more difficult to create and maintain sex symbols says former agent Steve Mather. "You have to work far harder because the media is much more fragmented and you have to make your mark as a sex symbol on all these individual magazines and TV channels."

Publicist Max Clifford says: "In the 1960s most of my experience was with pop and rock stars and you could get away with murder. I could say, for instance, 'The Beatles sold 50,000 albums this week' when they sold five. No one would check. I had no misgivings about making up stories because it gave the press something bigger and better to generate.

"It's hard to achieve and maintain a sex symbol's mystique today because everything moves so quickly and a sex symbol doesn't have time to evolve a persona in the way Connery and Newman were able to do. People are rediscovering them all the time. Also, we have a far more intrusive media and public.

"Nonetheless, it is possible to create a sex symbol, given adequate raw material. Let's say we have an attractive young guy who is in a major production, then it's not difficult even now to create a sex symbol mystique. The hard part is maintaining it, for the reality often is that he has very little charisma or self-confidence and hasn't a clue how to handle being a sex symbol.

"Sustaining an image is a marathon race not a sprint. You may have an initial boost – he is starring in *Four Weddings and a Funeral*, for example, and you can hype off the back of a hugely successful film. Then you gradually plant stories about your client in various parts of the paper. You let it be known that he helped a little old lady; it shows he cares. He must avoid appearing arrogant at all costs otherwise he won't last five minutes.

"Maybe we'll have someone else telling a story in one of the papers about what a wild, horny, incredible time she had with my client on some Caribbean beach. Or we'll suggest he marries so and so because he prefers boys and she prefers girls – it's a good arrangement – and they both look good together. So, when he does his next movie he'll still be a heartthrob and command $7 million.

"What's the truth anyway? I can take any newspaper today and read a lot of articles and think, 'well, we have a little substance here but that's a load of rubbish.'

"Trying to draw the line between reality and fiction is impossible. I have worked with stars and given them story lines and a year later they repeat them back to me. Then I have to remind them, 'Hold on, don't you remember? I made that up.'

"Sometimes they know they are lying but often they don't. We're not dealing in reality. It's virtual reality. It's infotainment – information as entertainment."

Footnotes:
1 From *The Hollywood Reporter, The Golden Years* by Tichi Wilkerson and Marcia Borie published by Coward-Mcann, Inc. Publishers.
2 From *Marilyn, Her Life in her Own Words* in collaboration with George Barris, published by Headline Press, London
3 From a TV documentary about Mel Gibson by Watchmaker Productions, presented and written by Clive James.
4 Ibid. 3
5 Taken from *A Woman's View, How Hollywood spoke to Women 1930-1960* by Jeanine Basinger published by Chatto and Windus
6 Taken from *The Hollywood Reporter, The Golden Years* by Tichi Wilkerson and Marcia Borie published by Coward-McCann, Inc. New York.

Through the Looking Glass

Star sex symbols are the elite in this age of celebrity. They inhabit a surreal world where fact, fiction and fantasy collide. We see them posing 'at home' in houses that have been borrowed for the photo shoot. We are given details of their inside leg measurement, the number of women they have slept with and the sexual positions they prefer. We read their fabricated life stories. Some of it may be fact, some it may not. But ultimately in this world of infotainment it is not important. What matters is to be true to the image, whatever the cost to the flesh and blood source.

The premier stars, aware that their continued success depends as much on savvy management as astute choice of roles, make it clear who is in charge, and with their great box office clout are able to wield immense control.

Kate White, Editor-in-Chief of Redbook, one of the most popular women's magazines in the US, commented on their power, saying: "I've not had to sleep with anyone, agent or publicist, to get a celebrity cover – yet."

Knowing that demand for information about them is at a premium, leading Hollywood stars can demand and get complete copy and photographic approval. This means they are allowed to read, vet and have the final say on what goes out about them in advance of publication.

Piers Morgan, Editor of the British Daily Mirror says: "I don't allow copy approval as a rule unless we're talking huge property. I'd have given it to Frank Sinatra just because having him talk to us would have been fantastic and I'd have given it to Princess Diana."

Being on the cover of a glossy magazine is more often than not a prerequisite of obtaining access to the likes of Tom Cruise and Julia Roberts – and is certainly not left to editorial chance. Moreover, should the interview take place, the odds are that a public relations person is likely to be sitting in on it to keep both star and journalist in check. Max Clifford's definition of a celebrity publicist calls to mind Svengali.

"You, the PR, are the person who often sits in on interviews, often tells them (the celebrities) what to say, often what to think. You are the person who creates the relationship. If you are about to interview celebrities it is worth bearing in mind that the PR knows more about them than anyone else, or should do, because if a star comes over here to do a film, say, you don't want any information coming out that is detrimental to them. I can, if I want, give wonderful exclusives to all kinds of people."

Richard Barber, a former editor of the British magazine OK, says: "If you try and organise an interview with an American star via one of their fearsome agents you are encouraged not to write one word of criticism – not unless you want to make it the last time you work with that agent.

"I know of journalists who have written film reviews for a particular movie and then have been barred by the studio from ever going to see any of their films because they dare to say the film is less than perfect."

If copy approval is an affront to every journalistic instinct, chequebook journalism is grounds for serious depression. According to media commentator Roy Greenslade, it dates back to the mid-1970s when the British newspaper The News of the World paid Christine

Keeler to retell her story, and The Sunday Mirror paid starlet Mynah Bird for what is believed to be the first kiss-and-tell feature. "It's now gone through the roof," he says.

Richard Barber concurs: "OK magazine bought the rights to Michael Jackson with his wife and first child – and they paid $2 million. It wasn't worth it in terms of what it did for circulation but you couldn't put a price on what it did to their standing. It indicated that they were serious players. So I think it was probably worth it.

"Newspapers used to pay more than magazines for stories but now they are outbid by Hello! and OK magazines which is why Fleet Street never misses an opportunity to take a pop at Hello whenever they can. You don't think 'hurrah', you just think, 'I've got a boss with a big chequebook.' I slightly deplore the way we have gone down that route."

Daily Mirror Editor Piers Morgan has no such reservations. "We make millions of pounds profit so why the hell shouldn't we get out our chequebook and buy properties that sell our papers? And celebrities are properties. They are in the public domain and if they've got something good they want to tell us and they want to make money out of it, fine. We are going to make money out of it too."

The trouble is there are simply not enough premier sex symbols to go round and so the popular press has created their own lesser-model variety. Emma Noble, entirely a media creation, says Morgan, is typical. As the fiancé of James Major, the former Prime Minister's son, a statuesque blonde, it suits the British tabloid press to pander to her desire for publicity.

"She looks the part and she latched on to a former Prime Minister's son which means she's news. She's good for us and we're good for her. It's probably quite good for James Major who has a stunning blonde on his arm which is something he would enjoy very much at his age. We get the benefit of putting them on the front page and people like reading about it. It's pretty harmless.

"But underneath it she may be a rather manipulative young woman who has set her sights on being seen with someone famous and getting in the papers. Are we joining in? Yes, we are to a certain extent. Does it matter? Probably not."

The Sun newspaper went so far as to invite their readers into the game. They wrote a piece admitting that they knew the event they were covering was merely hype for Emma Noble but they were happy to do it anyway. The underlying message was clear: she was so sexy and therefore so desired by their readers that it was worth colluding with hype, and then coming clean about it.

The much-vilified British tabloid press has developed a strange strain of schizophrenia in connection with their celebrity coverage. They are willing to pay many thousands of pounds for a 'must have' star feature (£250,000 is one of the highest sums The Sun admits to paying out) and submit to copy approval.

"I always give copy approval even when the celebs. don't ask for it because I don't want them vetting their own words," explains a leading tabloid feature writer. "My message is, 'Answer the questions honestly, I'll write it, you have a look at it and if you don't like it, I'll remove it.' We get a lot of flak about our handling of stories but with us, what you are is what you get." Such an approach, she says, has snared even Andrew Lloyd Webber, "not the kind of person you expect to see talking to the tabloids."

Copy approval is justified on the following grounds: it aids factual accuracy, very little copy is changed, and should it be cut, a partial interview is better than none at all.[1]

Whilst compromising on the feature pages, these same newspapers will deploy news reporters to dig up the dirt in an effort to bring down the stars. One such victim, says publicist Dennis Davidson, was Sly Stallone of *Rocky* and *Rambo* fame." In The Sun there was a three page spread on Stallone and a great film review. Fantastic. Then on a news page in the same paper there was this unsubstantiated story about steroids making him impotent. I don't know who the Editor was that day but it was totally ludicrous.

"You can understand why Stallone says, 'I don't want to be interviewed by these guys.' The British press now has the worst reputation the world. Trying to get talent to come here and talk to the tabloids is really, really tough. Because they will come and sit down with a show business correspondent and do a really responsible interview knowing that the paper he works for will pick up some crap about their lives a day or two later and make headline capital out of it."

This is but the latest tactic in the press' love-hate relationship with the stars, which has moved through three phases. First there was the sycophantic phase during the studio days when the journalist was in collusion with the star. The next phase was camped hostility between stars and the British tabloid newspapers that reached its nadir in the 1980s. "When I was on The Sun," recalls Greenslade, a former tabloid Editor, "you couldn't get a single interview with any star. Their agents and their PR's simply said no, no, unless the stars were up and coming.

"So we paid people for sneaky stories. But all the tabloids realised that they couldn't go on this way because they weren't getting enough personalities into their papers."

The cathartic moment was when Elton John successfully sued The Sun for libel and was awarded £1 million damages and a front-page apology. Piers Morgan, its newly appointed Bizarre pop columnist marked a complete change of tack. He was sent forth to become the friend of the stars and woo them with The Sun's four million circulation. Now Editor of The Daily Mirror, Morgan has been ideally placed to observe the transition from cold war to compromise, the third and current phase.

"Elton was so popular in the industry that absolutely nobody wanted to talk to us. So I had to get out there, go to parties, shmooze and be horribly charming and sycophantic to all the PRs and the agents who control this side of the business.

"Within six months we had gone from being on the outside to the inside by my saying, 'The Sun's going to change and if you want us to sell your film, album or book then you'd better get to like me. I for my part will guarantee that I won't turn on your celebrity act. Now the paper might do but I will always give you a more friendly platform.'

"It worked very well for a while but during my two last

years on Bizarre I was tougher because by then everybody

was prepared to talk to us. We would give celebrities a fair crack of the whip on interviews but we were far more critical of those who did naughty things. So we would constantly be falling out and making up."

The reason why the tabloid press and the public relations industry are so suspicious of each other is that they have completely opposite agendas. The main aim of the tabloids is to get a front-page lead out of a show business story and a scandal is the sure-fire way of obtaining it.

This, of course, is anathema to the publicists whose job it is to protect the image and reputation of their clients. "The bigger the star, the more time I spend keeping his name out of the media," says Max Clifford.

A major pop star who is caught brawling in a night-club is given two choices says Morgan. "We either expose him or we can agree a damage limitation deal where he might admit to x, y and z on condition that we leave out a, b and c. I've found if you play that game with celebrities about 90 per cent are appreciative and accept they have to be on page one. When that pop star punches someone out, the question is are we going to call him a monster? Or are we going to do a deal where he confesses to 'my shameful night, I'm so sorry.' It's all to do with the spin. I suppose we are glorified spin doctors."

It also has to do with what kind of celebrity they are.

"If you reach a certain level, you almost can't alienate the public unless you really handle it badly," says media commentator Greenslade. "Pop star Phil Collins divorced his wife by fax and no one felt too bad about Phil doing that – poor woman."

This is especially the case where the public accepts the persona as the person and blocks out anything that does not fit the image. When actress Sondra Locke wrote her kiss-and-tell book about Clint Eastwood, it did not sell well because, according to film academic Basinger, people had already made up their minds about him from seeing his films. As an icon, Eastwood's reputation is unassailable.

Although most sex symbols do not possess personas powerful enough to conceal or protect their real selves they may be pardoned their indiscretions if it is in keeping with their image. Rogue boys and rebel girls who are caught cheating, in flagrante, drunk or drugged may find it adds kudos to their wild and reckless reputations and in some instances make 'behaving badly' a professional policy.

Pop star George Michael's lapse in an LA public toilet was forgiven because it is regarded as acceptable for a long-established and highly rated singer-songwriter to be gay or bisexual. This would not have been the case had he been exposed when he was a member of the rock group Wham! (Wholesome, Handsome, Adorable Megastars!) and a teenybopper sex symbol.

Former Pop Music agent, Mather says: "Michael is obviously gay. But he would never have had a career at all if that had been known at the start because he was an idol. All the girls loved him. So he was always photographed with a girlfriend, never a wife because the fans wouldn't like it. Now it doesn't matter that he is caught loitering in toilets, he is credible in his field and no longer a sex symbol and so people are more tolerant. But had this incident happened when he was in Wham! It would have destroyed him."

The answer as to whether Aids victim Rock Hudson, who was the archetypal romantic Hollywood leading man, would have been able to have that career for as long as he did then, or at all nowadays is, however, by no means simple. According to film academic Basinger, it was no secret to the average American citizen that Hudson was gay. "I grew up in South Dakota which is as obscure as you can get. It's the fifth biggest state and the forty-ninth in terms of population. Yet I heard he was gay when I was in High School and Confidential magazine even carried the story in the 1950s. I remember my friend saying as we watched him in *All that Heaven Allows*, 'He doesn't look homosexual, does he?' But the way society was structured you did not go around blabbing about it all the time. The point is that if I knew it as a schoolgirl in South Dakota, how big a secret could it have been?

"It's the Anne Heche[2] question: When you know, does it change the way you see them? We are not sure of that answer and in Hudson's case it is complicated by the fact that he was the product of a studio system which groomed and promoted him, and no longer exists today."

Publicist Max Clifford is sure, however, that Rock Hudson could not have got away with his career intact today. "I know what is involved in keeping these things out of the media. Yes, people will accept the image but only if the real facts are not thrown in their faces as happened with Hudson."

He insists that there would be no licence from the public for Hudson the lover, who is publicly revealed to be gay. This would be in the same way that there is none for the teenage heartthrob who marries, or the leading man who says something out of turn about his co-star in a TV interview. They are all guilty of betraying the fantasy and they will be toppled.

Usually the press plays executioner. In public, people condemn the destructive stories and gossip in the media and demand a halt to intrusive paparazzi pictures and videotape footage. In private, however, they consume it avidly and then go into a state of denial. The obvious, though strangely unacknowledged truth is that our society is addicted to gossip and we find it shameful.

"Like smoking, it's not socially acceptable," says Greenslade. "Nobody who smokes will say anything other than, 'I really should give up.' And while they are in the act of smoking they will say, 'I shouldn't be doing this, I know it's bad for me,' but they are still doing it.

"The Princess Diana habit and the smoking habit are almost the same in the sense that we say, 'I know I shouldn't be reading this but I can't help myself.' Then we start rationalising it: one cigarette doesn't matter, one glimpse of Diana doesn't matter. But we are serially doing this and misleading ourselves. So we swear to give up reading anything about her.

"When we come to the act of purchase though, and it's a choice between five newspapers with big headlines about Diana and five without, we buy one with a Diana story. It doesn't do any harm, we say. It's only human nature."

Since Princess Diana's death, however, the press insist they are adhering to a revised self-regulatory code which aims to prevent the harassment and stalking of celebrities and to publish material that is in the public interest.

How then do they justify photographs of actress Farrah Fawcett Major swathed in bandages following plastic surgery, or of actor Tom Cruise's wife, Nicole Kidman leaving hospital after an operation?

"When celebrities are wheeled out into public streets and the photographer isn't harassing or pursuing, he just happens to be there, that's fair enough," says Editor Morgan. "Remember, these are celebrities who give endless interviews about their private lives. When Diana did the Panorama interview and revealed the most intimate details of her life I think she accepted she would be pretty fair game and subjected to scrutiny after that."

Morgan cites the refusal to use photographs of Paul McCartney in Paris walking with arms round his son, after wife Linda died as a prime example of how press policy has changed.

"The papers would have definitely published those photographs five years ago, no question. They would have made page one. But nobody used them after Paul McCartney's agent said he really rather we didn't because he felt they were intrusive and that Paul wouldn't like it."

I have a sneaking suspicion also that the British public would not have appreciated it either. McCartney might be an overwhelmingly famous pop legend and have been knighted, but through his actions and behaviour – staying out of the limelight, taking the occasional bus, going to the local cinema – he still manages to come across as a regular bloke, a real human being. Equally, his relationship with Linda was perceived as real and so there was a genuine public desire that he be shown the courtesy and respect due to a man who had lost his dearly beloved wife – and be allowed to mourn in peace.

This could not, of course, be in greater contrast to the public's attitude towards the death of Princess Diana. She ceased to be regarded as purely human long ago and when the people mourned, they were mourning an icon.

The public has become so familiar with the screen images and personas of its chosen sex symbols that it feels it knows the people upon whom they are based – and what is more, that it has the right to own a piece of them. 'We made them what they are. They owe it to us,' is a commonplace attitude.

There is an increasing sense that they exist for our pleasure and that by being public figures they forfeit their private lives. If they do have them, however, their private life is our business as much as theirs.

The X-Files actress Gillian Anderson says: "It angers me when pictures are taken of me together with my daughter. I have had a lot of people tell me, 'If it bothers you, then get out of the business.' But that can't be right. That isn't the answer."

Psychoanalyst Margot Waddell at London's Tavistock Clinic says: "The idea that because these stars have this incredibly glamorous life, they owe us in some way is a terribly interesting one. What makes some people think they may be entitled to somebody else's life or success? The subject has been very little addressed in the psychiatric profession and we've got to try and understand it because this feeling takes people out of their own skins and makes them feel they are part of an identity that isn't their own. Such people have developed a false conscious-ness."

The feeling of entitlement may have its seeds in a grad-ual blurring of reality and fiction. Media commentator Greenslade says: "You can have relations with people on TV that you don't have with people in real life. It's far easier to do that and involves less commitment – and you can go and do something else the minute you don't fancy doing that.

"Switch on the TV, see a star, star dies. Switch on the tears. Easy. For you are in control of all those emotional situations when you are dealing with someone remote from you, whereas when it's someone close to you, it is far more difficult and painful. "Remember the man at Princess Diana's funeral who said he wasn't able to cry when his wife died but cried when Diana died. There you have the classic example of somebody substituting an unattainable figure he didn't know on to whom he could pour out his genuine feelings, rather than exhibit those feelings over someone he knew and presumably loved – extraordinary."

An added factor is that some viewers may actually spend more time watching and relating to their favourite soap and TV stars than they allocate to friends and rela-tives and so feel they know the fictional characters better than their real Aunt Jane in Liverpool.

"Some people act as they know me," says actress Gillian Anderson. "It's interesting – if they are yelling at me from across the street they'll call me by my charac-ter's name. But those who approach me call me by my name. Some people are completely nervous, some even break down in tears.

"I've got used to these sorts of reactions over the years. A lot of people are surprised to see how normal I am, how normally I dress. Occasionally somebody is obsessive, yes. I diffuse the situation by being nice and showing the person behind the obsession that I am also a human being."

THE AUDIENCE VIEW

Leonardo DiCaprio is the answer to pubescent girls' prayers around the globe and the level and intensity of fan worship is overwhelming proof that sex symbols mean more to this age group than any other.

But while so many of their parents are resigned to the Leo obsession and the media have written reams on the subject, they admit that they find his appeal inexplicable.

'Bland' and 'unlikely' are adjectives that might be used in connection with his features, along with those typically bestowed on first-class dreamboats: poet's brow, cherub lips and ocean-blue eyes.

Indignation abounds. This isn't Cary Grant/Clark Gable/Harrison Ford but a mere boy-child of an actor, they splutter. How on earth can he be a sex god? Feminist Camille Paglia went so far as to describe him as looking like a 13 year old lesbian – unwittingly she has summed up his appeal.

DiCaprio is the latest and most successful example of the Pretty Boy type that has always enthralled the pre-teens and teenage girls. He is the male version of their best friend and distinctly unthreatening. His androgyny is his greatest asset. It makes him safe.

The global hysteria he has induced is, ironically, a phenomenon that is based on the avoidance of sex. For these women-to-be, DiCaprio is their fantasy first boyfriend.

By choosing him as a model for future romances they can effectively stonewall the whole issue of sexuality and emotional relationships in their lives. By seeing or feeling themselves in a relationship with him they are working out how they should respond when attracted to somebody, and how they would want that person to respond to them.

Journalist and best-selling author Celia Brayfield, says: "In both sexes, I suspect, when sexuality first bursts through into life, the kids are actually looking for someone who is very like them. Adults who are disturbed by the androgynous appeal of these adolescent sex symbols miss the point that their audiences are seeking an outward personification of their own sexual confusion. It follows that they will identify with a public image in which these qualities are not distinct."

They are characteristically products of the pop world; sensational commercial success and passionate fan worship mark their brief existence.

Counselling was offered to hundreds of distraught fans after the group Take That split up. Some even took action by marching on Downing Street and delivering a petition to No.10 asking the Prime Minister to intervene.

Media Production student, James Abrehart worked for MTV as part of his work experience and observed: "There were lots of competitions to go on a date or meet the pop stars backstage but you had to be 18 or over to enter.

"Nonetheless, we'd get mail from fans all over Europe asking us to tell Peter Andre that they loved him and would we contact him on their behalf. Their letters rarely included their ages but judging by their handwriting and the naivety of what was written I'd say they were between the ages of 13 and 18 years. They went for very handsome grown-up or not so grown-up boys in celebrity boy bands. After Take That split up, the three most popular groups were The Back Street Boys, Boyzone and East 17.

"I was also involved with organising the small audiences who came to watch the pop groups and film stars being interviewed live and again, although the official line was 18-25 years only, very often kids a lot younger than that turned up." My own very informal survey[3], in which I persuaded 41 people of both sexes, aged between from 13 to 63, to fill out a questionnaire, showed that three-quarters of them had chosen a pretty boy singer or teenybopper band as their first sex symbols. The rest picked pretty boy actors and actresses. They ranged from Kylie Minogue, Aaron Carter and The Back Street Boys at the young end of the spectrum to Tommy Steele, Cliff Richard, The Bay City Rollers, the young John Travolta and the exceedingly popular David Cassidy (who reflected the high number of female respondents in their late-30s and 40s) at the other.

Hairdressing assistant Joyce Attree who was a teenager when the films *Saturday Night Fever* and *Grease* first came out, says: "We all wished that our lives could be like theirs; taking off in cars, caring for each other, suddenly singing. But most of all we thought 'cor, wouldn't it be great to be able to dance like that or go a dance club like that.' It was a fantasy teenage life."

Denise Robinson, a one-time avid Cassidy fan, recalls: "He was a very romantic figure, the kind I would have liked as a boyfriend. His appeal lay in his voice and he had this look which would melt you. When you are 15 you think you are in love and to me he was a god. All my friends felt the same.

"I once spent a whole day at Heathrow waiting for him to come through. When he did, we screamed and went mad with hysteria. I remember being amazed – I didn't think I would be like that. My claim to fame was that I actually touched his arm – and I almost fainted.

"Going to a David Cassidy concert was like a grand group day out. The train into White City was full of Cassidy fans and we'd painted his name on our hats, scarves and even our heads. I even had 'David' sewn into my bra. One girl had a Cassidy tattoo done and I thought that she would live to regret it. Big fan though I was, I did suspect it was a passing phase.

"The concerts didn't start until 8 or 9.00pm but we would get there in the morning because the build-up was important. Together, we queued and we sang his songs – we all felt we shared a common bond.

Robinson was exhibiting typical teen behaviour in her adoration of Cassidy. What was unusual is that she had a serious boyfriend whom she married at the age of 17. "I was engaged to Steve while I had this passionate crush on David Cassidy. But I was always able to separate reality from fantasy and although Steve thought I was over the top, he accepted that I came with David Cassidy. Of course, I thought the whole fan thing was normal because all my friends were going through it too.

"When I got married and moved away from home I couldn't take the posters with me but I did keep them in the loft for a long time. I still have some of his tapes and out of nostalgia I play them now and again.

"I remember seeing him on TV a few years ago, and some of those 'he's nice' feelings came back as I was watching it.

"I still think he is a talented performer but when he got married I went off him, even though I married about the same time. All his fans thought he had betrayed us, because at 15 you believe that you are going to meet him and marry him. The fantasy can be broken very easily. I am sure that a lot of Cliff Richard's evergreen popularity is due to the fact he has never married."

Psychoanalyst Waddell believes fan worship, to a certain extent, can serve an important function for adolescents "who are all over the place: terrified about their own bodies, want to look good but feel awful. And who at the same time are struggling to come to terms with the terrifying issues of who they are, of losing their childhood, of facing an unknown future and wondering whether they will ever find someone to love them.

"One way of avoiding the feeling that 'no-one understands me,' 'I'm different from every body else,' 'I'm completely alone,' is to find temporary reassurance in figures such as DiCaprio. 'Everyone understands me because everyone my age loves DiCaprio and understands why I love DiCaprio.' So I feel that some of these escape routes from the difficulties they confront in their internal world have a developmental function, provided they don't become an essential ingredient.

"The danger is that they may cling to a fantasy or visual image rather than developing their own internal capacities because they feel that the two-dimensional attachment is more reliable and manageable."

Awareness of sex symbols can start as young as 6 years of age owing to children's unprecedented exposure to the mass media and may be incorporated into their play. Sophie Holdsworth, now aged 11, learnt the following rhyme at school when she was 7 and taught it to her then 6 year-old-sister Emily:

My name is Elvis Presley, Girls are sexy
Sitting in the back seat drinking Pepsi
Watching the movies
Pinching boobies
Having a ballsy in the Navy
Boys blow kisses
Girls go whooo!

(as they exclaim, they lift up their skirts)

Sophie progressed to The Spice Girls and her parents spent almost £100 on a family trip from Cambridge to see the band in concert at Wembley. When Geri Halliwell left, Sophie cried because she thought the group would split but by then both girls had discovered Leonardo DiCaprio.

Interestingly, their fascination for DiCaprio arose without them even seeing the film *Titanic*. "I was regarded as the meanest mother on earth for not taking them to see it but it was rated a '12' and they were too young. However, it didn't stop them from buying one of his biographies and a poster. Sophie is currently saving to buy the video of *Titanic*," says Sue Holdsworth. "She's quite realistic though. There's no, 'Wouldn't it be nice to go on a date with Leonardo DiCaprio?' She's far more interested in real boys at the dance studio we attend.

Di Caprio by no means appeals only to pubescent girls. A considerable number of women in their late thirties and forties relish his boyishness that reminds them of young men they knew in their youth. Sue Holdsworth says: "Obviously torrid passion is not the appeal here. He makes you want to cuddle him, to look after him. Another person who falls into this category is Anthony Edwards in *ER*. "I have always preferred him to George Clooney because you want to make it alright for him. He's got that little boy lost appeal and there is something of that in DiCaprio too."

Equally, older women are seduced by the character of Jack played by DiCaprio in *Titanic*. One experienced female publicist says: "I think every woman would like to be treated the way Jack treated the heroine Rose."

And the escapist appeal of his bohemian existence should not be underestimated either. Holdsworth says: "There's a line in the movie where he says he gets up every morning not knowing where he will be sleeping that night. That element is very appealing when you live a very ordered routine existence.

"It offers the possibility of difference, the possibility of casting aside ties and responsibilities. You don't necessarily want that something else, you are not necessarily discontented with what you've got but the option is there. I don't think your life need be deprived to appreciate this form of escapist fantasy. You could live a luxurious and fulfilled life but still the grass is always greener and watching DiCaprio is a harmless way of indulging it."

Young boys are much more into body parts – mechanical as well as female.

They are preoccupied with machismo and male sex symbols that they can emulate. My nine year old son Christian and his friends are typical in having James Bond as their hero, played by Pierce Brosnan.

John Newberry, 11 years old when interviewed, showed me a room dominated by cars, football teams and anonymous models advertising bras and pants he had cut out of mail order catalogues. A magazine picture of a swimsuit clad Pamela Anderson paled into insignificance beside his poster of footballer Ryan Giggs.

"Pamela Anderson is my favourite pin-up because of her figure and she's blonde. I'm probably too young to go out with girls but I would like to go out with someone like her.

"I don't think of the girls at school in the same phwoah way. Some of them are my friends, so you don't think about their looks. I like them for their personality and I think women should go for your personality, too. But I have to admit I am not going for Pamela Anderson's personality so I am being slightly hypocritical."

Morgan Floyd-Walker, 16, believes that the male sex is more realistic in their appraisal of sex symbols.

"You see women crying when they see their idol at a

concert. We just think, 'She's a bit of alright.' I used to fancy Meg Ryan until I was 14 but after seeing her in a film I wouldn't think about her, or talk about her, whereas girls I know will have long conversations going 'cor.' I don't think it goes that deep for men. Women will buy pop magazines like Just 17 – men don't bother. They'll buy a CD instead.

"All of us at one stage or another have put up posters on our bedroom walls because it's nice to look up and have something beautiful to see. The human form is really attractive to look at – that's why sex symbols are used to sell everything, everywhere."

And the truth is that sex symbols need not even be alive to do. The 'must watch' car advertisement of 1998 starred a resurrected Steve McQueen, the king of cool in the 1960s. In a high-tech film splicing operation, the car McQueen had actually been driving in the film *Bullitt* was cut away and replaced by a silver Ford Puma.

Then the original drive scene through San Francisco was mixed and matched with film from a modern day shoot. A reference to one of the star's other major movies, *The Great Escape*, was also made when McQueen pauses and passes a motor bike.

Surrey hairdresser Rosie Brown says: "It worked because Steve McQueen's image suited that car. He gave it a sexiness." Her assistant Joyce Attree adds: "Every time that ad was on I'd sit down and watch it. Actually I'd watch Steve McQueen in anything, over and over again. He gives out such a strong sexual aura. It's his look and the way he turns round. He's like Paul Newman. They both have those eyes." Indeed, eyes, smile, warmth and approachability are the main criteria upon which women, aged 21 and up, judge male sex symbols.

Harrison Ford scores highly overall, and according to a January 1999 survey by the American magazine US is the star most American women would like to date.

"Looks alone won't do it. They've got to be approachable and Harrison Ford is a sex symbol you can imagine in carpet slippers," says Surrey publican Linda Walaszkowski. "He seems like a nice person – very relaxed and comfortable with himself, but not showy. He is someone who would know how to make you feel at ease. The roles he plays reinforce that image. I've also seen him on chat programmes, which allow you to see a star in a different light. I think you see more, or think you are seeing more of the person behind the image."

But surely, I countered, a professional and experienced film star like Ford could act nice just as he could act any other role.

Walaszkowski argued that whatever the actual truth, the reason Ford is so successful is because his nice guy image is perceived as being an extension of his personality.

"The difference between stars and actors is that the star's personality always comes through. Sean Connery is always Sean Connery. Mel Gibson is Mel Gibson and Harrison Ford is always Harrison Ford. As far as I'm concerned the roles fit them, they don't fit the roles."

Ford is the personification of the modern-day male sex symbol. Unlike Newman or Gibson who possess "those eyes," he neither possesses an exceptional physical feature, nor is he astonishingly good-looking.

He is, however, the ultimate ordinary guy star who has been elected by us to have the kind of adventures of which our dreams and nightmares are made, and to undergo an extraordinary variety of trials and tribulations which must be overcome in a manner befitting a human hero.

Human is the operative word here. Ford is universally popular because he is the star with whom we are most able to identify – someone, not too unlike ourselves, whom we can imagine wearing carpet slippers.

The ancient Greeks would have recognised him instantly as the mighty but very human hero, Odysseus. The wandering warrior who spent ten years fighting monsters and witches, evading sirens and enchantments before he reached home. 'Of all mankind,' Athena the goddess of wisdom tells Odysseus in the Odyssey, 'thou art easily foremost, both in counsel and speech.'

He was her favourite and he is ours too. Whether he comes in the guise of Hans Solo or Indiana Jones, the beleaguered assassin in *Blade Runner* or the bewildered cop in *Witness*, he epitomises the wisdom, shrewdness and heroism man is capable of – without Superman's tricks or Bond's special effects.

Conversely, remote and enigmatic stars are out of favour. They are perceived as cold, not cool, and their self-containment is easily interpreted as arrogance or narcissism. For make no mistake, arrogance is the great unforgivable sin against which liaisons with prostitutes and loitering with intent in public loos pale into insignificance, and any celebrity found guilty will be toppled in a trice.

"They can't be too sure of themselves. I have an aversion to these sex symbols who are in love with themselves," says beautician Carol Tilbury.

Even those in the business are not immune from showing bias towards the more accessible star, as can be detected from publicist Patric Scott's comparison of Warren Beatty's sex appeal with that of Mel Gibson.

"Mel Gibson was a really nice, open guy with wonderful warm sexiness that shone out. It captivated everybody. Take that, project it on the screen and you have a great force. Contrast this with Warren Beatty who came on to the set when I was working on *Yentl* years ago.

"In terms of looks he had it all. Everybody thought he was dazzling. But his beauty and his image were very, very remote. It was 'look but don't touch.' Beatty seems to be in an ivory tower. Consequently he is not so acceptable on the screen as Gibson who is much warmer, affable and approachable."

Beatty is considered less appealing because he does not bow to his audience. He does not publicly concede that he needs us and we feel a touch spurned.

Linda Walaszkowski says she ceased to be a fan of his when she saw him being interviewed on TV about his film *Dick Tracy*. "He made unflattering remarks about Madonna, his leading lady. I was very disappointed. He came across so high and mighty."

Yet audiences are equally capable of behaving in a high-handed manner and we have a history of being notoriously fickle to boot. We judge our celebrity sex symbols differently from ourselves and our neighbours.

American journalist Elsie B.Washington says: "Take DiCaprio, for instance. Questions have been raised about his sexuality and I am sure it would affect his box office power if it were ever categorically proven that he is gay. This has no bearing on how we feel about gays in general – they may be our close friends.

"But when it comes to a fantasy figure, someone who is supposed to be our idol, then gays are not acceptable and we are ruthless and contemptuous in our dismissal of them as romantic leading men."

Even when sex symbols fulfil the highest expectations of their audience, it is no guarantee of loyalty as Ailsa Rea, a 22 year old zoologist is the first to admit. Tom Cruise, her first pin-up, had all the qualities she insists upon in a sex symbol.

"He must have the perfect face, the perfect body and the perfect personality – well, maybe not the personality – not so much. But he must have the look: not a hair out of place, perfect muscles and no blemishes."

Nonetheless, she cast him aside because he got older, to be replaced by Patrick Swayze and John Travolta in quick succession. At the time of interview her heart-throbs were Brad Pitt whom she would go and see in anything, and TV actor Dean Cain who plays Superman. But they are probably already history – particularly in Cain's case, for Rea was never that keen on Superman's flying suit. While the approachability factor is crucial in a modern day sex symbols' appeal, it may be applied in varying degrees and the audience can be divided into two distinct groups.There are those who imagine inviting their heartthrob in for tea and a cuddle and visualise him as their ideal husband and then there are those who prefer to preserve a little distance and simply have them 'just there' to look at and admire. Sex symbols who satisfy the former are Harrison Ford and George Clooney; Paul Newman and Brad Pitt, the latter. Mel Gibson and Sean Connery manage to appeal to both sets.

Jayne Miller, a lifelong moviegoer and passionate autograph hunter in the late 1970s has observed the gradual reduction in unattainability.

"I was brought up on Errol Flynn, Gary Cooper and Tyrone Power movies, and stars such as Olivia de Haviland, Vivien Leigh and Hedy Lamarr were far more unattainable than actresses today because they were so glamorous. They were never seen looking ordinary.

"Seeing a star in the flesh was a thrill but it also had the effect of making them attainable. They don't have the same presence because you are no longer able to see the character they were laying on stage. Take away the character and you've just got the man. They even look smaller than when on stage. Image is everything and I think stars are more constrained by their image today. In the old days they were given a greater variety of roles for the simple reason that they made many more films than today.

"Essentially though I don't think the appeal of sex symbols has changed. Even in our society of allegedly open and available sex, when you look up on the screen and see Mel Gibson the average woman knows she will never meet that type of man. He is a fantasy, so you sit there and drool.

"Sometimes the fantasy is a little frightening, different from what we would go for in real life. You wouldn't necessarily want to marry someone like that. I mean if I met Martin Riggs, Gibson's character in *Lethal Weapon*, I'd run a mile. It goes right back to seeing what you don't have or wanting what you can't have – it shows ideal possibilities.

"Perhaps the star on the screen reminds you of good times you have had in your life and by watching them in a movie you can recapture some of it in your imagination. You can fantasise about whatever you like at a basic level or on a romantic level.

"Mystery is as important as it ever was. Those of the old school such as Sean Connery know how to retain it. So does Mel Gibson despite being a modern actor. They don't divulge everything. The Clive James TV interview with Gibson was fascinating because it was clear you were only seeing what he wanted you to see.

"We watch these star interviews in the hope that we might get an insight into the real them but I think we are more or less happy with the image because that is what we ultimately want to see – that's what being a sex symbol is all about.

Female sex symbols are judged by men on their 'phwoar' factor, which predictably is contingent on their good looks. But while "massive boobs, lovely bum and shapely legs" figured prominently in the male interviewees' conversations, more than half also found the faded jeans, baggy jumper, and hardly any make-up look "very sexy."

"If you can look sexy in that, then you really are sexy," says 23 year old Sam Butler. Former agent, Mather concurs: "For many men my age, the actress Felicity Kendall mucking around in an Aran sweater, digging up potatoes in the TV series *The Good Life* is the ideal."

While Cameron Diaz and Sandra Bullock were at the top

of the list for men in their late teens and early 20s, those in their late 30s and 40 s frequently mentioned older women in their 50s such as actresses Joanna Lumley and Francesca Annis.

Interestingly, Annis who became a sex symbol when she played a TV version of Lily Langtry is perceived as all the more alluring because she is living with *The English Patient* star Ralph Fiennes who is some 13 years her junior.

Women over 21 who judge female sex symbols on their natural beauty, vulnerability and resistance to the ageing process chose Liz Taylor and Goldie Hawn as their ideal older woman sex symbols. "I take my hat off to Liz Taylor, the way she keeps coming back after all her illnesses, and managing to look glamorous," says Joyce Attree.

Rosie Brown, 22, says of Hawn: "She's so natural. I'd love to look so good when I'm her age. Her body is exceptional. She might have had tucks but it doesn't look as if she's had anything done."

It used to be that a star could simply "put on her face" to go out and meet her public. But obvious make-up no longer signals sex appeal or glamour – rather it is seen as something false, a cover up. The aim is to look natural and to achieve it, female sex symbols are going under the knife for plastic surgery as a matter of course, and nipping and tucking in record numbers. And so are their male counterparts, who realise that their audiences now take sculpted pecs and rippling arm and leg muscles for granted. Our sex symbols show the extent to which ideal beauty, inextricably linked to sex appeal, has reverted to the ancient Greeks' vision of perfectly sculpted bodies – only this time round, women are included.

Footnotes:

1 Journalist Heidi Kingstone conducted a 2- hour interview with Maurice Saatchi for the Mail on Sunday. Copy approval regarding his quotes had been agreed. He cut all but one line. The newspaper ran the article without Saatchi's deletions a month later with Kingstone's consent. Kingstone argued it was unreasonable for Saatchi to give such a wide-ranging interview and then expect the article to run with almost no quotes.

2 Actress Anne Heche was publicly and controversially revealed as Ellen's lover after Ellen admitted she was a lesbian in the U.S TV comedy sitcom of the same name.

3 see appendix II

The Future

The shape of sex symbols to come may well be influenced by one of the most potent sex symbols of the past – Marlon Brando. He wants to be immortalised through digital technology and become the world's first virtual actor.

"Marlon is a consummate computer artist and has been keeping an eye on the progress of synthetic actors and environments since the beginning of the industry. So we decided he should be the first synthetic actor," says Scott Billups, a cyber-evangelist who has pioneered digital production for film, TV and virtual actors in Hollywood. Brando and Billups rented a small jet and flew up to the Cyberware facility in Monterey, California, which developed and houses the machine that digitally records the human subject's features. "We spent a day scanning Marlon into the computer. The data set was so dense that it took almost a year to refine it into a presentable form."

The conversion of flesh and blood Brando as we know him today into a virtual reality model of his youthful self has a surreal quality about it. Access to the elusive fountain of eternal youth, it seems, is by way of a glorified barcode scanner. The signs of age are swept away but the resulting image is not the iconically beautiful Brando face that we are familiar with. Yes, it is a youthful version of the older man but it is altogether different from the young Brando. The nose is hawkish rather than aquiline, the cheek bones more pronounced, the lips thinner and slightly drooping at the corners and the face more angular. There is a fleeting resemblance between the actual and virtual reality young Marlon images. But the true likeness is between Brando senior and the virtual reality model.

The before and after pictures, with the two faces side by side, look like father and son and demonstrate the process known as 'age morphing.'

For although technology makes it possible for Brando to look youthful, it is as yet unable to recapture the way he used to look because it can only work from the data provided by his face and features as they are now.

"The face is by far the hardest element to work with," says Billups. "There is little difference between the synthetic body types. But we are so keyed to the subtle nuances of motion in the human face that the slightest transit can convey a wide range of emotion. For this reason there are more control points in the faces of our characters than in any of the dinosaurs in *Jurassic Park*.

"Instead of a laser beam merely sweeping across the item, as with a barcode scanner, the Cyberware Scanner sweeps around the object being scanned – in this case, Marlon's head. We scanned his face numerous times while he formed different expressions and vowel sounds," explains Billups.

Once the library of scans was completed it was necessary to correlate the data. For instance, the thousand points of information that comprised the left eyebrow needed to match throughout the thirty or so various scans that comprised their library of "facial variables." The same exhaustive and time-consuming work was entailed in correlating the cheeks, the nose and then the lips until all of the points on the face were systematically connected. The better the correlation, the better the results.

The implications of a Virtual Marlon are far reaching.

Theoretically, Brando could act behind his youthful, synthetic image and become a sex symbol the second time around even though he might actually be in his late-70s. He could be an eternal franchise of himself.

Brando tested the immortal possibilities in the early 1990s when he had Billups scan his face for an hour-long TV documentary that featured his actual, senior self interviewing a very early virtual version of his younger self. Beside the latest virtual Marlon, the prototype is primitive but it showed Hollywood that synthetic actors, commonly known as synths, could do more than stand in for sick or injured stars.

"As far as stars are concerned, it will allow them to work on several roles at one time," says Billups. "A synth never needs cosmetic surgery and never gets sick or old unless the role calls for it. They can play any role, at any age, in perpetuity. What could be better?"

Forrest Gump director Robert Zemeckis illustrates this graphically. "Imagine having Brando today playing Stanley Kowalski[1]. He would perform, and all that emotion, all that style and all those moves would be his, but his physical presence would be manipulated by the computer or enhanced by the computer. Instead of having young actors putting on make-up to look old, he could be an older actor looking young."

This is by no means pie in the sky, sci-fi speculation. Brando looks set to collaborate on a feature length movie, Software, for Phoenix Pictures, to be directed by Billups. Based on a sci-fi novel of the same name by Rudy Tucker, the plot concerns the subjugation of free will as a society of lunar robots tries to absorb the minds of humans, a variation on the theme of the endless search for the soul. Billups intends creating about eight hundred synthetic characters for this project.

He has his work cut out for him. Much of the synthetic work he has done in movies is concerned with special effects, where the 'synth' has been on screen for only 20 or 30 frames at a time, usually standing in for an actor during a dangerous stunt. "More recently I've been getting requests for characters that will eventually command their own roles."

He insists that audiences will "buy it" because they already accept a film industry that is built on synthetic situations occurring in synthetic environments. "Many dialogue scenes in movies are shot with only one actor. The person that they are having a conversation with is usually in a trailer watching soaps. Human-synthetic interaction is not a problem."

However, if we accept that an actor's quintessential talent is to persuade us that the feelings he generates on the screen are genuine, even though we know he is only acting, then the interaction between a virtual Brando and his audience becomes more complex, because we know his 'self' as well as his emotions are fabricated.

Billups disputes this, saying: "Whether the image is recorded directly from the organic original, or created from a data-set that was previously gathered from the original, who cares?

"I think our idea of what constitutes a sex symbol is up for re-definition. Heck, I thought Jessica Rabbit[2] was a babe. Forget suspension of disbelief, sex appeal is in the context. Rather than focusing on the past, I'm looking to current projects to help re-define what is sexy."

Just how synths 'emote' and thereby provoke emotional responses in their audience has less to do with chemistry than computer technology. "There are a dozen major physiological functions that represent the emotional and physical response in the human body. By classifying and cross categorising various emotional expressions we can quite easily create a 'fast-learn' subroutine."

His creation of a virtual Marilyn Monroe is absolute proof, if any were needed, that an authentic sex symbol is more than the sum of her body parts.

"Part of the process included casting sessions for body parts that were duplicates of the real Marilyn. Ears, eyes, hands, body-type; in fact, just about every part of the real Marilyn was duplicated in our casting. These 'parts' were then scanned into the computer and used to create our synthetic representation."

GTE Interactive, the company which commissioned Billups to create a fully articulated Marilyn Monroe to promote an upcoming movie release of *Life After Death* supplied him with three of the top Marilyn Monroe doubles who were scanned at Cyberware and made history. Theirs were the first full body data sets created on Cyberware's recently completed vertical scanner.

"We did several motion capture sessions with Susan Griffiths, considered to be the leading Marilyn impressionist, which translated Monroe's classic gestures and nuances into binary code. The various inflections that she incorporates into her range of motion is quite evocative of the former organic Marilyn."

Once the physical form had been roughed in, work started on hair, clothes and motion. Surprisingly, one of the hardest elements to create convincingly on the computer is, well, hair. "The hardest part for us was the digital hair styling," says Billups. "The hair is essentially straight and must be gathered in groups and curled. Curls and hair groupings are then given a degree of flex, bounce and elasticity which will eventually add up to a realistic appearance.

"As we discovered when we started assembling and scrutinising Marilyn's physiology, she was really quite average – almost dumpy, even by 1950's standards. Her feet and ears were enormous and her hands were anything but glamorous.

She had a bulbous little nose that reminded me more of Karl Malden than the sex goddess she was supposed to be. What the heck was going on here?

"When we finally had created a geometrically accurate Marilyn and rendered her out we thought that there must be something terribly wrong. This couldn't possibly be the geometric form of mankind's ultimate sex symbol.

"It wasn't until we applied the surface texture (make-up) and motion that she really started to become recognisable. A test we did of Marilyn standing still and looking directly into the camera did not rate as high as a test we did of a 'walking-talking' Marilyn. I guess it isn't the looks as much as the moves that make us sit up and take notice – kinda like a fishing lure."

The digitisation of stardom has divided Hollywood. A number of leading stars have asked for limits on the presence of digital images in their movies. In 1992, ABC World

News Tonight carried a piece on synthetic actors in which director Robert Wise described Billups' work with synthetic actors as 'bastardising the industry.' Tom Cruise has since made speeches to fellow directors and actors warning of the dangers. These include competing with virtually resurrected stars and possibly even pornographic virtual versions of classic stars.

The economics of film making, however, will see to it that synths will inevitably play an increasing role. "Actors have long been the most undependable and expensive components in the conventional story-telling scenario while synthetic actors are tireless artisans of limitless potential. Synths based on real organic persona stand a good chance of taking over an ever-increasing share of the industry," argues Billups.

"The potential for syndication of the synthetic persona is even more extraordinary than that for the persona of a real star. Look at how attached we have become to our stars' personal lives and thoughts. Just walk into your local bookstore and count all the books by celebrities.

"Secondly when you place your synth into a virtual location they are really there. The degree of presence is unlike anything that we can create with conventional production technology. There is an undeniable trend towards interactivity yet no one can make it work using organic actors. For real interactivity we are going to need synths who can adapt and react to an unimaginable number of probable scenarios.

"Like it or not, synthetic characters are our future. As the analog generation dies off and the digital generation comes into power I believe we shall see a steady shift from the carbon bias to the inorganic. Science fiction, who knows? We might as well get started now."

Which brings us to science fiction writer William Gibson's novel Idoru.

'Idoru' is Japanese for idol, a term which Gibson appropriated for his digital heroine. But the twist is that this virtual idoru gains an actual consciousness; it expresses a desire to merge with a human admirer. The admirer, a world famous rock star has prolonged his star status by using a digital image of his youthful self.

Since he wrote that book we have seen the emergence of Kyoto Date, the world's first virtual reality pop singer and the even more ubiquitous virtual reality sex symbol Lara Croft. Who knows, they and their kind could provide a way out for our reluctant human sex symbols?

In place of our human pantheon of sex gods and goddesses we could establish a virtual reality Mount Olympus in the knowledge that these digitised sex symbols, always available yet unknowable, would be able to interact with their audience on a one-to-one basis, anytime, any place – without the risk of invasion of privacy, or intrusion.

According to Billups, within two or three years we shall start to see organic personalities emerge from these virtual reality models and within four or five years we can expect them to demonstrate a basic capacity for synthesised original thought. A first step, perhaps, on the way to the Bladerunner replicants?

Moreover, their images would be physically perfect, last forever yet at the same time offer the promise of constant change because of their mutable composition. If this sounds familiar that's because it is. These are precisely the qualities possessed by the Greek gods and goddesses of old which their followers simply called divine.

Footnotes:

1 Brando's charismatic performance as the male lead Kowalski in *A Streetcar Named Desire* earned him an Oscar nomination in 1951

2 Jessica Rabbit was a cartoon blonde bombshell in the feature film *Who Framed Roger Rabbit?* starring actor Bob Hoskins who seemed rather impressed by Jessica too.

Appendix

The rare film poster market is very volatile but it can be lucrative.

Value is based largely on scarcity and many popular posters are rare, even if thousands were printed when the film was first released. Posters accompany the movies they promote as the films travel from cinema to cinema. When the run is over, the film and the posters are put in storage. When the warehouse is full, the posters are generally destroyed to make more room.

Consider that of the 8000 original posters issued in America for *Breakfast at Tiffany's*, starring Audrey Hepburn, only about 300 remain in existence. The surviving posters are worth in excess of £1,800.

Serious collecting of cinema posters started about 16 years ago. In the early days, the posters produced in the 1960s and earlier were available for a few pence. Now they can change hands for hundreds or thousands of pounds.

Sotheby's, London and Christie's, South Kensington, have poster auctions in September, and The Reel Poster Gallery in London's Great Marlborough Street carries a selection of classic British and international posters.

Popular posters and their current prices (all in excellent condition) include the following sex symbol posters: *Le Mepris*, 1963, starring Brigitte Bardot – £800; *Thunderball*, 1965, starring Sean Connery as 007 – £500; *Au Bout de Souffle*,1959, starring Jean-Paul Belmondo – £450; *Moon over Miami*,1941, Betty Grable and Don Ameche – £6,750; *The Graduate*, 1976, starring Dustin Hoffman and Ann Bancroft, 1967, – £500; *The Sting*, 1974, starring Paul Newman and Robert Redford – £175; *A Hard Day's Night*,

1964, starring The Beatles – £750.

APPENDIX II

The informal survey forms were completed by Surrey customers and clients of Studio 56 Beauty Centre, Beare Green, Sebastian's Hairdressers, Elarose dress shop, Dorking and 14 year old members of a Surrey football team, The Roffey Youth F.C., Horsham.

The most striking finding was the popularity of Elvis Presley and Marilyn Monroe among the 20 - 29 year olds, comprising 11 females and one male. Four nominated Marilyn Monroe as the ultimate sex symbol of this century (3 females, 1 male) and three nominated Elvis Presley (all female). Presley was selected for his singular good looks, "swoon making" singing voice and sex appeal; Marilyn Monroe for her looks, curvaceous figure, real life intrigue and above all, her vulnerability. Sean Connery appealed to four females, all of whom liked him as 007 (one has liked him since the age of 8 years).

No icons featured in the 14 - 18 age group but "sexual personalities" dominated. Denise Van Outen, Kate Winslet and French actress *Beatrice Dalle*, of Betty Blue fame were popular but three males nominated Sam Fox as the sex symbol of the century because they regard her as the ultimate Page Three pin up.

Marilyn Monroe and Sean Connery were the overwhelming choice for ultimate sex symbol of the century for the 33-39 year olds, with Paul Newman as a possible contender. Mel Gibson, Harrison Ford and Jamie Lee Curtis were named as popular sex symbols.

An almost identical picture emerges among the 41 - 45

year olds who regard Marilyn Monroe and Sean Connery as their sex symbol of the century. The difference is that this age group likes Connery as he was and as he is today. "His sex appeal has not decreased with age," says a 45 year old female respondent.

Harrison Ford and Mel Gibson (female choice) and Goldie Hawn (male and female choice) are the most popular sex symbols.

Apart from the 63 year old female respondent who voted for Charles Bronson and Clint Eastwood, all the others voted for sex symbols much younger than themselves. One 51 year old female respondent included DiCaprio, Christian Slater and Brad Pitt in her list of favourites.

This group in general demanded good looks as well as personality in their sex symbols. Ralph Fiennes, Pierce Brosnan and Richard Gere were especially popular, and in their twenties and thirties their favourites were Connery as Bond, Robert Redford and Tom Cruise.

Again their teenage choices reflected their penchant for good looks: Gary Cooper, Errol Flynn, Richard Chamberlain (beauty combined with bedside manner in *Dr. Kildare*), and Cliff Richard.

What is particularly interesting is that apart from the teenybopper and pop groups and singers, all respondents selected their sex symbols from film and TV, although one 26 year old male respondent did list Margaret Thatcher as someone he considered a sex symbol when he was 17.

Quiz

ARE YOU A GOD, (OR A MERE MORTAL)?

Answer the following questions as honestly as you can. Note down the letters which are in brackets after each answer you have chosen that you feel most closely reflects how you are. Sometimes the same letters will appear after two different answers, but this does not matter.

1. Get your kit off, take a look at yourself in the mirror, and what do you honestly see?

a) A devastatingly handsome fellow – basically drop dead gorgeous – I must remember to admire myself more often, I'm such a lucky chap. (D, AP)

b) A fit, toned and strong body – ready for action – of any kind! (HL, O, AR)

c) The latest version of whichever image I am portraying at the moment. (HM)

d) A boyish, (or younger than I really am) body. (E, AD)

e) Started off well, but too much good living is not doing me any favours! (D)

2. How do women see you?

a) As a wise and fair man, who also happens (luckily) to be very handsome. (AP)

b) As a charmer, whom women find irresistible. (AR, D, AD, E)

c) They admire my physical strength. (HL)

d) As a hero/action man. (O, AR)

e) They never really know me – I constantly re-invent myself. (HM)

3. Do you feel you have a feminine side to your nature?

a) Yes. (D, HM, AD, E)

b) No. (HL, AP, AR, O)

4. Do people seek your advice and counsel on life's problems?

a) Yes, often. (D, AP, HM, O)

b) Not really. (HL, AR, AD, E)

5. Which statement most accurately reflects your outlook on life?

a) I believe in playing fair and will always seek out the truth. (AP, AR, AD)

b) In life you play to win; and if that means a few untruths, or a little unpleasantness along the way, then so be it. (HM, O)

c) I'm very good at persuading other people to do what I want them to do. (D, E, HM)

d) I get very angry and sulk when things don't go my way. (E, AR)

e) I like to be the centre of attention. (HL, E)

6. What is your attitude towards women?

a) They are there for my pleasure and delectation, and I take every opportunity to sample their many delights. (D, HM)

b) They are very much the opposite sex – I love them but I cannot claim to understand them. (HL, AR, AP)

c) I feel they are friends as well as lovers – I can relate to them on any level.
(O, D)

d) I admire and feel very comfortable with women – I often enjoy spending time with women more than I do with other men. (E, AD, D)

7. Would you say you are:

a) Always ahead of the game in most spheres. (HM, D, HL, O)

b) An excellent team player. (AP, AR, AD, E)

8. Your interests lie mainly in which arena?

a) Business, finance, the commercial world. (HM)

b) The arts and entertainment. (D, E)

c) Sport, action and adventure. (HL, AR, O)

d) Science and discovery. (AP, AD)

e) Law, society, truth and justice. (AP)

9. Which statement applies best to your nature?

a) I am very competitive and prefer to lead. (HL, AR)

b) I am very creative and individualistic, I like to go my own way. (D, HM, O)

c) I go with the flow and work best alongside others. (AD, E)

d) I prefer to keep my own counsel and I trust my own judgement. (AP)

10. What would you most like to be remembered for?

a) My professional achievements. (HM)

b) My sex appeal and my romantic conquests. (AD, E)

c) My sporting or action adventures. (HL, AR, O)

d) For being a loving, family man. (O, D)

e) My ability to constantly reinvent myself, and surprise and amuse others. (HM)

f) My wisdom and fairness.(AP)

11. You know your body best. Are you a natural mover? How do you most like to spend your spare time?

a) Taking part in any active sport – football, swimming, dance, athletics, hockey, riding, and making love energetically (with plenty of grace and passion!)
(D – SHS, HL, AR, AD, O, AP)

b) Watching sport, sitting at my computer, propping up a bar, reading, painting / drawing, and making love with a minimum of energy (but plenty of sensuousness!)
(D – SC, E, HM, AP)

12. Which group of characters in the public eye do you most admire and identify with?

a) Jack Nicholson, Michael Douglas, Gerard Depardieu, Gary Oldman.
(D, SC)

b) Richard Gere, John Travolta, Patrick Swayze, Tom Jones. (D, SHS)

c) Arnold Schwarzenegger, Sly Stallone, The Gladiators. (HL)

d) Paul Newman, Robert Redford, Michael Jordan . (AP)

e) David Bowie, Julian Clary, Michael Jackson, Steve Coogan.
(HM)

f) Tom Cruise, Harrison Ford, Mel Gibson, Kevin Costner, Pierce
Brosnan.
(AR – AM)

g) Andre Agassi, Michael Jordan, Michael Owen. (AR – GS)

h) George Clooney, Johnny Depp, Brad Pitt, Kiefer Sutherland.
(AR – R&R)

i) Tom Hanks, Steve Martin, Robin Williams, Dudley Moore. (E)

j) Leonardo DiCaprio, Ewan McGregor, Keanu Reeves. (AD)

k) Harrison Ford, Denzel Washington. (O)

SCORING.

Count up how many times each letter or group of letters appears in your score.

The more frequently each letter or group of letters occurs, the more similar you are to each god or mortal.

Check below to see where your true godly or mortal nature lies!

MOSTLY D'S, D – SC'S, D – SHS'S.

You are Dionysus, half mortal, the god of dance and ecstasy. Yet you are also the only god, who, once he found the woman he wanted, was totally faithfull. You have a snake personality. You are determined, ambitious and cagey. You are very interesting to others, subtle in your ways, and you think deeply. You may also have a very beautiful voice.

In questions 11 & 12, you will have noticed some additional letters after D. If you chose D – SC, you are a Snake Charmer. Very intelligent and creative, you can also be very opinionated. You know exactly how to make a woman feel good, and you are also loyal to your own sex.

If you have a weakness it is a tendency to do everything to excess.

If you chose D – SHS in questions 11 & 12, you are a Snake Hip Seducer. You have an amazing, almost mesmerising sex appeal. You are so well co-ordinated you have an almost panther-like way of moving. You are capable of great grace and could be a professional dancer.

Your weakness could be a tendency to abuse others, taking

advantage of your immense sex appeal to lure them into your trap!

MOSTLY HL'S.

You are Hercules, the strongest man. You really enjoy pumping iron and enjoy your body both looking and being masculine, strong and fit. So long as your woman believes you are God's Gift, you will go to the ends of the earth for her.

You are strong and brave, and a defender of women. You will always rescue a woman out of a tight spot!

You tend to feel you have to work for what you get, things don't come easily.

You are not stupid. You understand the value of your assets and you use them. Other people tend to underestimate you, you are cleverer than people give you credit for. Sometimes you capitalise on this.

Your weakness is a need to be the centre of attention.

MOSTLY AP'S.

You are Apollo, the god of truth and justice. Not only are you damn gorgeous, you are clever too.

Naturally, you tend to be a role model and inspiration to others. You are certainly a real man, nothing boyish about you. You are responsible, faithful, caring, you have gravitas, you can be selfless, you know how to cherish women.

You want a woman as a companion and partner, an intelligent woman, as well as an attractive one.

You are very persistent - you never give up. Your weakness is that you can be intractable and obdurate at times.

MOSTLY HM'S.

You are Hermes, the god of new beginnings, motion and commerce. You have a chameleon nature. You are always changing.

You always look different in photographs. You are very aware of fashions and trends, and you embrace these. Sometimes you are ahead of the game, which you enjoy. You love ideas and playing around. You can have a very airy-fairy side to your nature, but you are always shrewd with money. This does not mean that you are not very generous to your friends, you are. But you also make sure that you invest and save when you can. You are also clever with words, and will lie quite happily. You have an extraordinary degree of self-confidence, you are brazen, almost to the point of shamelessness. Rarely will you get embarrassed.

Your main weakness is a tendency to stir things up and cause trouble.

MOSTLY AR'S.

You are Ares, the god of war. You are very physically fit and take a pride in your appearance. Even if you abuse your body because of your tendency to addiction, you seem to have a constitution of iron. You love being outdoors.

In question 12 if you chose AR – AM, you are an Action Man. You are individualistic, not a team player. You have a tendency to eccentricity and like going your own way. You think on your feet. You also cut your losses and start again easily. Any girlfriend of yours can tag along to what you want to do if she feels like it. You like your lover to share your interests, and to have interests of her own too, not so that you can join in, but so that she won't mind when you disappear off to do your own thing.

If you chose AR – GS, you are a Great Sport. You are very much a team player. You are competitive, determined, and you want to win.

You have to achieve in life to feel content.

If you chose AR – R&R, you are a Rebel & Rogue. The ultimate charmer, you can get away with murder. You are also unreliable, brooding, a loner, and want to go your own way. When women are with you they feel wonderful, you are such fun to be with. But the trouble is, they never really know where they are with you.

You have dark, menacing side to your nature.

MOSTLY E'S.

You are Eros, the cupid god of love. You might actually be (or have been), quite a pretty young man, and people will often think of you as cute. You are very sweet natured and nice. You can also be very clever, and you will listen and be sympathetic to others. People will feel comfortable with you and confide in you.

You can make people laugh and they enjoy your company.

But because your childlike personality often comes to the fore, you can also be obdurate, manipulative, persistent and mischievous.

Because of your insecurity, you care too much what other people think.

You have a tendency to be a very dependent person. Basically, you need to grow up and develop greater confidence.

MOSTLY AD'S.

You are Adonis, a mere mortal, but a beautiful, youthful one. You cannot help but know it, of course, women go mad for you. But you are not a shallow character. You enjoy your looks, but you want women to like you for more than this. You are not irresponsible, and if you are fickle, it is simply because you are young.

You do still have a teenage personality, you can be moody, but also funny, strong and confident. You want a partner, and you will feel better when you are married.

If things go right for you, you could turn out to be an Apollo.

MOSTLY O'S.

You are Odysseus, another mere mortal, but again, a gorgeous and clever one at that. You are a hero adventurer, a swashbuckler, a risk-taker, and a romantic. You cherish your women. You are a genuinely nice young man, sincere, chivalrous, and caring. To you, women are very much the opposite sex. You celebrate your own masculinity, and you love women for their femininity. Before you settle down, you might do your share of womanising, you are so romantic and warm you tend to fall in and out of love easily.

You will always be a bit of an adventurer at heart.

ARE YOU A GODDESS, (OR A MERE MORTAL)?
Answer the following questions as honestly as you can. Note down the letters which are in brackets after each answer you have chosen that you feel most closely reflects how you are. Sometimes the same letters will appear after two different answers, but this does not matter.

1. OK now be honest! When you look at yourself naked and unadorned in the mirror, what do you really see?

a) A voluptuous, womanly, bountiful beauty! (AP, HL)

b) A slim, girlish body. (HB – W, AR, E, HM)

c) A gorgeous, sexy babe. (HB – M, HL, HB – W)

d) A strong, fit body. (AR, AT, HM)

e) An ordinary body with good and bad points. (AT, E)

2. When you were a teenager at school, who were you more popular with?

a) Boys. (AP, AR, HL)

b) Other girls. (AT, E)

c) About equal. (HB – W, HB – M, HM

3. Do you feel you have a masculine side to your nature?
a) Yes. (HM, AR, AT, AP – A)

b) No. (HB, E, AP – E, AP – I, AP – F, HL)

4. If you were going to be cast in a role for a film, which role would you be able to play best?

a) The romantic, glamorous lead. (AP)

b) The loveable and funny girlish character. (E, HM)

c) The scheming manipulator. (AP – I, HM, E)

d) The intrepid adventuror. (AR, AT, AP – A)

e) The mother figure. (AP – E, AP – F)

f) The clever career woman. (AT, HM)

g) The passionate sexpot. (HB – M, HL, AP – E, AP – F)

h) The helpless waif in need of rescuing. (HB – W, E)

5) As a child, (and the child in you now), which activities did you prefer?

a) Outside – climbing trees, exploring, making up adventures, playing with your dog. (AR, AT, AP – F, AP – E, HB – M)

b) Playing games at home – dressing up, playing with your dollies and teddies, stroking your cat. (E, HM, HB – W, HL)

c) Painting, drawing, making things. (HB – W, AT, HM)

d) Plotting your next strategic move in board and card games. (HM, AT, AP)

6. If you wanted to get your own way with a man, any man for any reason, which strategy would you be most likely to adopt?

a) Burst into genuine, heartfelt tears. (E, HL, HB – M)

b) Work out exactly what his problem/perspective was, and devise a clever argument to counter his.
(AT, AP – E, AP – A, AP – I)

c) Shout, scream, rant and rave, turn on the crocodile tears if necessary.
(AP – F, HBW)

d) You almost always get your own way. Men seem to fall over themselves to please you. (AR, HL, E, AP)

7. Would you almost rather die than be seen out in public without make–up and clean, groomed hair?

a) Yes. (HL, HB – W, E, AP – F, AP – I)

b) No. (HB – M, AR, AT, AP – E, AP – A, HM)

8. Are you basically a very warm personality?

a) Yes. (AP – F, AP – E, HB, HL, E)

b) No. (AP – I, AP – A, AR, AT, HM)

9. How do you relate to men?

a) I love them. Men are some of my best friends, as well lovers. (HB – M, AT, AP, AR, HM)

b) I find them confusing but I need to have one around. Can't always live with them, but can't live without them either. (HL, HB – W)

c) I need a man to take the lead. (HL, E)

d) I tend to relate to them mainly on a sexual level. (AP – E, HL)

e) I really enjoy, and feel more comfortable in men's company. I've always been more like one of the lads. (AR, HM)

10. Are you the type who would leap into the sea naked for a midnight swim, or some such other joyous and impulsive activity?

a) Of course! Things like that are usually my idea anyway! (HM)

b) Only with my best boyfriend. (E, AP, HL)

c) Perhaps if I was tipsy and dragged in by my friends. (HB)

d) No way. I'm far too sensible for such nonsense. (AR, AT)

11. What would you most like to be remembered for?

a) My magnetic, knock-out effect on men. (AP)

b) My professional achievements. (AT, HM, AR)

c) My unpredictability and creativeness. (HM)

d) My warm, generous and humourous personality. (E, HB – M)

e) My sporting / dancing / athletic achievements. (AR, AT)

f) My beauty. (HL, AP)

g) My kind, caring, and nurturing personality. (AP – E, AP – F)

h) My wisdom and sense of fairness and justice. (AP – I, AP – A)

12. What's your biggest fear?

a) Losing control. (AT, HB – W, AR, E)

b) Not having a man around. (HL, AP)

c) Being bored. (HM, AT, AR, HB – M)

d) Losing my looks. (HL, AP)

13. Which group of characters in the public eye do you most admire and identify with?

a) Kate Moss, Courtney Cox, Jennifer Aniston. (HB – W)

b) Kate Winslet, Cameron Diaz. (HB – M)

c) Diane Keaton, Gillian Anderson. (AT)

d) Jamie Lee Curtis, Sigourney Weaver. (AR)

e) Demi Moore, Madonna. (HM)

f) Goldie Hawn, Felicity Kendal, Meg Ryan. (E)

g) Sophia Loren. (AP – F)

h) Susan Sarandon, Ellen Barkin. (AP – E)

i) Catherine Deneuve, Grace Kelly (AP – I)

j) Michelle Pfeiffer, Gwyneth Paltrow. (AP – A)

k) Pamela Anderson, Jane Fonda as Barbarella (HL

SCORING.

Count up how many times each letter or group of letters appears in your score.

The more frequently each letter or group of letters occurs, the more similar you are to each goddess, or mortal.

Check below to see where your true goddess or mortal nature lies!

MOSTLY HB'S, HB – W'S, HB – M'S.

You are Hebe, the goddess of youth. Your natural build tends to be very slim, girlish and fragile, you look like you need protecting. You may have a tendency to be obsessed with diets and being thin, perhaps verging on the anorexic, imagining you're overweight when you're not.

If you chose mostly HB's / HB – W's, you are Hebe, Waifs & Strays.

You are very charming and disarming, and tend to be liked more by the opposite sex than your own.

You are also fashion-conscious, materialistic, and very stylish.

You do know your own mind, but you tend to be rather insecure at times, and feel that you need a partner who will take care of you.

Luckily, men who will see your physical fragility will also feel that they would like to take care of and look after you!

Naturally, you sometimes use this to your own advantage. You might play the little girl, but you are actually very ambitious, and strong underneath.

Because of your insecurity, you are also rather secretive about your real feelings and needs; there is a part of you which no-one else knows.

You do revel in lots of attention and feel much happier if you are the centre of attention.

You are actually a much stronger person than you think you are, and you would be wise to remember that.

If you chose mostly HB's / HB - M's, you are Hebe, Millenium Eves.

You are a slender young beauty, and all the boys want you, lucky girl! You are more confident in yourself, and you do have a fun personality and a more happy-go-lucky outlook on life. Essentially you are well-balanced, secure and direct in your interactions with others. You enjoy your good looks (who wouldn't?), but you scarcely give them a passing thought at times, you are more interested in just enjoying life and finding out what it has to offer you. You realise you are very blessed and very fortunate, and things just seem to come easily to you. You are very popular, and have many friends.

You are ambitious and prepared to work very hard, but you don't show it.

To others, your achievements seem to happen with almost effortless ease!

MOSTLY AT'S.

You are Athena, battle goddess of education and science.

You are fit and alluring, the cleverest of all, and the most power-ful. Your cleverness comes from both you innate ability, common sense, and from your naturally curious nature. You are very wise, and will happily offer your wisdom and advice to those who seek it, not in a dogmatic fashion, but subtly. Sometimes, if the person is not listening carefully, they might miss hearing your wise words, which is a pity because you really do know what you're talking about. They are fools not to listen.

You are always more clever than your opponent, you think several moves ahead, and you would make an excellent lawyer. You love ideas, but sometimes you are so clever you use them in an amoral way.

If you love someone you invest all your emotions in them and get fully involved.

You have a strong nurturing side and will look after your man and support him in every way – you are such an asset to have as a partner, because you help your loved ones to fulfil their potential.

On the downside, you can be selfish and preoccupied with your own ideas. You would make a very bad enemy, people are unwise to oppose you as you will make trouble for them.

MOSTLY AR'S.

You are Artemis, goddess of wild things, dance and hunting! You are tomboy woman. You are independent, clever and fit. You have a directness and an honesty about you which is very appealing. A naturally joyful and happy person, people like being with you, and always feel better when you're around. You are very quick in your nature and abilties, and don't suffer fools gladly. You could be superwoman, you are capable of juggling many things at the same time. You can easily be one of the boys. Men really like you, they also respect and admire you – you are rather intriguing to them!

You are quite athletic, it is important to you to work out and keep fit. You care about your body and want to look after it.

You are very well co-ordinated, both physically and mentally.

You're not one for glitz. You prefer unobtrusive elegance.

You are a very sensible and dependable woman, and a good friend to have.

MOSTLY HM'S.

You are Hermes, goddess of new beginnings, motion and commerce. You are an intellectual; clever, very aware of what's going on around you and very adaptable. You love change, you seek it out and you embrace it, you are like a chameleon; you change your colours to suit your mood. You are so confident that you don't really care what others think, you are happy to go your own way, say your own thing, be brazen, be upfront, be shameless, if it suits you to be so. What a mischief-maker you can be!

At your worst, you will lie quite happily, and stir up trouble for others if it amuses you or suits your purpose. You just love ideas, and playing around to see what will happen.

At your best, you are inspiring, creative and ahead of your time.

MOSTLY E'S.

You are Eros, cupid goddess of sweethearts! You are so pretty and cute (you may have dimples) , you can get away with quite a lot of mischief if you want to! You are not malicious, but play-ful, and great fun to be with. People enjoy your company because you are not competitive or challenging. This is not to say you lack ambition. If you set out to achieve something, you think it through carefully and persist in your efforts to get it. This usually results in a high level of success. You are gentle, sympathetic and understanding; you are a very soft-hearted and warm person. Because of the 'sugar' in your personality, people can underestimate you – they shouldn't, because you have plenty of spice too!

You are also quite childlike at times, and if you don't get your own way you are very hurt. You simply can't understand how people won't always do what you want. This frustration makes you stubborn and obstinate. You may also then start to become very manipulative and persistent in order to get your own way. You cry easily, but you can soon be comforted and cheered up by a kind phrase, a warm smile, a twinkling eye and a big hug. People can soon put that lovely smile back on your face again!

MOSTLY AP'S, AP – F'S, AP – E'S, AP – I'S & AP – A'S.
You are the Ultimate Divas, Aphrodite, goddess of love and beauty. What a woman! Because you most definitely are a woman, and not a girl. You look womanly, your shape is curvaceous, you have all the womanly physical attributes of breasts and hips and bottom. You are a naturally sexy and uninhibited person. Men often place you on a pedestal, which you tend to find rather amusing as you certainly don't place yourself on a pedestal.
However, you do have a very strong personality, once you have thought carefully and made up your mind about something, you are unlikely to change. All this can frighten any fellow who isn't a real man! (You would certainly know how to turn a boy into a man, if you can't find a real man to be with!)
Your colouring may be golden and glowing, or dark and mysterious.

Mostly AP – F's – you are a Fire Diva. Your nature is fiery and unpredictable and you like it that way. You love to keep others guessing. Of course you are warm, your temper is quick to flare up, and equally quick to die down. You are a spontaneous person, and if you are self-disciplined you have a great capacity to keep a number of tasks on the go at the same time.
Your downside is that you can roar into action in a very OTT way and kill things off before you realise what you've done.

Mostly AP – E's – you are an Earth Diva. You are naturally down-to-earth; sensible, practical, and passionate in a very earthy way. You have an innate cheerfulness about you which is very attractive. Your personality is very well-balanced and 'grounded'. People who feel insecure or upset love to talk to you because you make them feel grounded too. You're easy-going, and are happy to go with the flow.

You are very sexy and capable of reducing a man to a quivering jelly!

Mostly AP – I's – you are an Ice Diva. You are so cool, people find it hard to get close to you or understand you. You're self-contained and very much in control. But anyone who gets through to you will discover your white heat!

But first, people have to prove their worth to you. You are not passive but contained, and put potential friends and lovers through their paces. In searching for your soulmate, you will never compromise or accept second best. You are not after looks. It is your own personal assessment of a person's traits that you trust, and by which you are guided. You are very confident and comfortable with your own decisions and values, and any potential suitor would have to meet with all your requirements.

Once you find your man, he will never think of you as ice again! This is because your ice is a defence mechanism, to mask your vulnerability. You will melt in front of him once he has passed all the tests you have set for him.

Mostly AP – A's – you are an Air Diva. You are a very elusive woman, men who meet you may feel that it could take a lifetime to tease out all your possibilities. You work hard and become very skilled and accomplished at whatever you set out to achieve. You manage to make your accomplishments appear effortless. You are trustworthy. Your airy nature means you need space to do your own thing, you must be allowed this freedom, then your are more than happy to come back home. You will be very faithful and perhaps have many unorthodox and platonic relationships with men. An exceptional Diva, you are equally popular with both women and men. You tend to be minimalist in your dress, possess an innate grace, and you will always look young, even in your eighties and nineties.

MOSTLY HL'S.

You are a mere mortal, Helen of Troy. But what a babe! You are beautiful and value this asset highly. You are an upfront, in-your-face kind of girl. You are really great fun, and you are honest. You ooze (and use) your sex appeal to get your own way, and are overtly ambitious. This can get you on the wrong track if you're not careful. You need to use it in a classy, and not a vulgar way if you are not to get exploited.

Because of your youth and your physical charms, to you your sex appeal is a commodity to be exploited. Your youth makes you very vulnerable to men, who may prey on your combination of innocence and beauty. Men love you, but you are not the most popular girl on the block with your own sex. Take care while you are growing and maturing not to be too reckless and foolish.

When you mature you may grow up to become one of the four Aphrodite Divas.

The Family Tree of Principal Sex Symbol Archetypes

Gaia - Earth

Uranus - Heaven

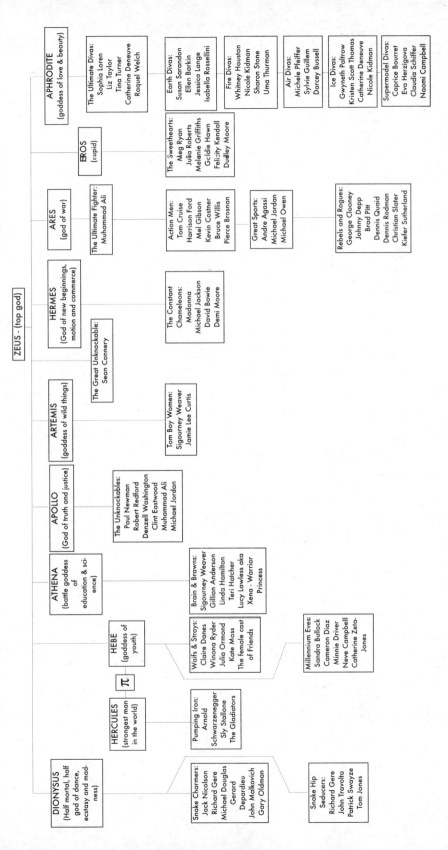

The Family Tree of Principal Sex Symbol Archetypes (cont.)

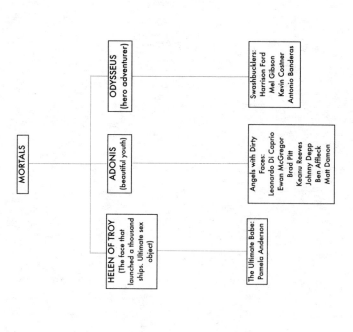

MORTALS

HELEN OF TROY
(The face that launched a thousand ships. Ultimate sex object)

ADONIS
(beautiful youth)

ODYSSEUS
(hero adventurer)

The Ultimate Babe:
Pamela Anderson

Angels with Dirty Faces:
Leonardo Di Caprio
Ewan McGregor
Brad Pitt
Keanu Reeves
Johnny Depp
Ben Affleck
Matt Damon

Swashbucklers:
Harrison Ford
Mel Gibson
Kevin Costner
Antonio Banderas

Index